Patient Care

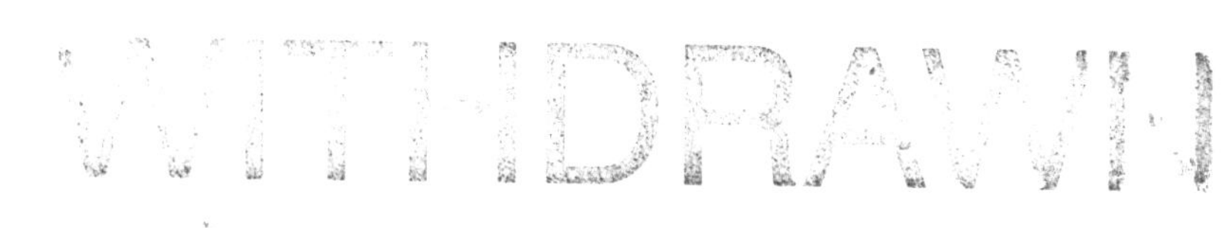

NOTICE

Medicine is an ever-changing science. As new research and clinical experience broaden our knowledge, changes in treatment and drug therapy are required. The author and the publisher of this work have checked with sources believed to be reliable in their efforts to provide information that is complete and generally in accord with the standards accepted at the time of publication. However, in view of the possibility of human error or changes in medical sciences, neither the author nor the publisher nor any other party who has been involved in the preparation or publication of this work warrants that the information contained herein is in every respect accurate or complete, and they are not responsible for any errors or omissions or for the results obtained from use of such information. Readers are encouraged to confirm the information contained herein with other sources. For example and in particular, readers are advised to check the product information sheet included in the package of each drug they plan to administer to be certain that the information contained in this book is accurate and that changes have not been made in the recommended dose or in the contraindications for administration. This recommendation is of particular importance in connection with new or infrequently used drugs.

Patient Care

ERICA KOCH WILLIAMS, M.Ed., R.T.(R)(M)

Assistant Professor of Allied Health
Medical Diagnostic Imaging Program, Allied Health Department
Fort Hays State University
Hays, Kansas

SERIES EDITOR

STEWART C. BUSHONG, Sc.D., F.A.C.R., F.A.C.M.P.

Professor of Radiologic Science, Department of Radiology, Baylor College of Medicine, Houston, Texas

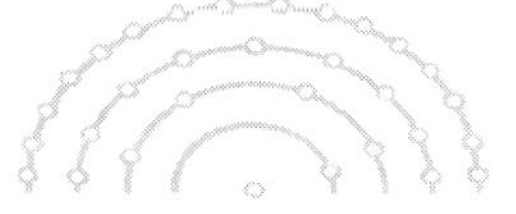

ESSENTIALS OF MEDICAL IMAGING SERIES

McGraw-Hill
Health Professions Division

New York St. Louis San Francisco Auckland Bogotá Caracas Lisbon London Madrid
Mexico City Milan Montreal New Delhi San Juan
Singapore Sydney Tokyo Toronto

McGraw-Hill

A Division of The **McGraw-Hill** *Companies* 

PATIENT CARE

Essentials of Medical Imaging Series

1 2 3 4 5 6 7 8 9 0 MALMAL 9 9 8

ISBN 0-07-070632-8

This book was set in Berkeley by V&M Graphics.
The editors were John J. Dolan and Peter McCurdy.
The production supervisor was Heather A. Barry.
The text designer was José R. Fonfrias.
The cover designer was Robert Freese.
Malloy Lithographing, Inc. was printer and binder.

This book is printed on acid-free paper.

The forms on pages 3, 120, and 126 are used courtesy of Sunnyside Community Hospital, Sunnyside,Washington.

The photos on pages 12 and 13 are used by permission of JT Posey Company, Arcadia, California.

FirstTemp Genius© Tympanic Thermometer photos (p 18) provided courtesy of Sherwood-Davis & Geck, St. Louis, MO 63103.

Filac© F-2000 Electronic Thermometer photo (p18) provided courtesy of Sherwood-Davis & Geck, St. Louis, MO 63103.

Standard Precautions signage (pp 35, 36, 38, and 42) is reproduced by permission of Brevis Corporation, 3310 South 2700 East, Salt Lake City, Utah 84109, 801 466-6677.

Visit The McGraw-Hill Health Professions Website at http://www.mghmedical.com

Cataloging-in-Publication data is on file for this title at the Library of Congress.

Contents

Preface

This book is part of the new McGraw-Hill series, Essentials of Medical Imaging. Stewart Bushong, as Series Editor, is the brains behind the concept for this series and I am pleased to be working with Stewart on this book.

Patient Care is intended primarily for the student but faculty should find it a useful supplement to their teaching. Quality patient care is the foundation of our science and the information in this volume should be viewed as the core concepts in patient care. In addition, the design of the book facilitates a better understanding of facts. The combination of illustrations and short statements is unique and provides the students with better tools for an examination.

At the end of each chapter there are practice questions patterned after the respective qualifications examinations, such as the ABR, the ABMP, ARDMS, the CNMT and especially the ARRT and its subspecialty exams in mammography, computed tomography, angiointerventional procedures and magnetic resonance imaging. Most exam panels principally use Type A questions and those are the majority of the questions here.

There are three appendices at the end of this volume. Appendix A is a substantial glossary of terms employed in patient care/imaging sciences. Appendix B lists appropriate textbooks for further study. Appendix C contains the answers to the questions.

Patient Care is the foundation of Medical Imaging as well as other sciences. Though health care may change, high quality patient care should not, and I hope this book provides a better understanding for the student.

ERICA KOCH WILLIAMS

Acknowledgments

This book would not have been possible without the support and contributions of my family, friends, and colleagues. I would like to thank Jennifer J. Fitzgerald, Richard Thomas Rossmeisl, and Sean Patrick O'Flinn for offering their time, critiques, and knowledge. Their honesty, expertise, and humor were much appreciated.

My sincerest gratitude to my editor, John Dolan, who was a constant source of patience and composure. I praise his ability to smooth my feathers. Bob Lapsley, the illustrator of this work, truly performed miracles with what little my artistic abilities could provide.

Principally, I wish to thank my family for their encouragement. Publicly I must recognize my parents, Janice Furtado Koch and Henry Stephen Koch, for their sacrifices, faith, love, and support, which will shape my life forever. To my siblings, Stephen, Susanne, and Hy, I love you for letting me be your sister and friend. Finally, my daughter Elyssa, to whom this work is dedicated, you make my true purpose evident.

Dedicated to

Elyssa, may the eyes of your understanding always be open to truth and knowledge.

Patient Care

American Society of Radiologic Technologists
Code of Ethics

1 The radiologic technologist conducts himself or herself in a professional manner, responds to patient needs and supports colleagues and associates in providing quality patient care.

2 The radiologic technologist acts to advance the principal objective of the profession to provide services to humanity with full respect for the dignity of mankind.

3 The radiologic technologist delivers patient care and service unrestricted by concerns of personal attributes or the nature of the disease or illness, and without discrimination, regardless of sex, race, creed, religion or socioeconomic status.

4 The radiologic technologist practices technology founded upon theoretical knowledge and concepts, utilizes equipment and accessories consistent with the purpose for which they have been designed, and employs procedures and techniques appropriately.

5 The radiologic technologist assesses situations, exercises care, discretion and judgment, assumes responsibility for professional decisions, and acts in the best interest of the patient.

6 The radiologic technologist acts as an agent through observation and communication to obtain pertinent information for the physician to aid in the diagnosis and treatment management of the patient, and recognizes that interpretation and diagnosis are outside the scope of practice for the profession.

7 The radiologic technologist utilizes equipment and accessories, employs techniques and procedures, performs services in accordance with an accepted standard of practice and demonstrates expertise in minimizing the radiation exposure to the patient, self and other members of the health care team.

8 The radiologic technologist practices ethical conduct appropriate to the profession and protects the patient's right to quality radiologic technology care.

9 The radiologic technologist respects confidences entrusted in the course of professional practice, respects the patient's right to privacy and reveals confidential information only as required by law or to protect the welfare of the individual or the community.

10 The radiologic technologist continually strives to improve knowledge and skills by participating in educational and professional activities, sharing knowledge with colleagues and investigating new and innovative aspects of professional practice. One means available to improve knowledge and skills is through professional continuing education.

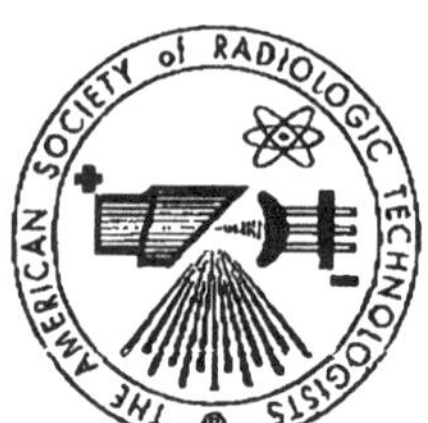

Revised and adopted by The American Society of Radiologic Technologists and The American Registry of Radiologic Technologists, July 1994

Legal and Ethical Responsibilities

CHAPTER 1

STANDARDS OF PRACTICE

- Radiologic technologists (RTs) are governed by a **Code of Ethics** and **Principles of Conduct** established by the American Society of Radiologic Technologists (ASRT) and the American Registry of Radiologic Technologists (ARRT).
- The Code of Ethics serves as a guide for professional conduct evaluation.
- The **Scope of Practice** defines specifications for RT responsibilities.
- Patients are protected by the **Patient Bill of Rights**, established by the American Hospital Association, which details distinct expectations of the patient as a client of a health care facility.

ETHICAL CONCERNS

- **Ethical issues** are based on moral responsibilities and values.
- **Values** are derived from numerous sources to include one's culture, experiences, and religious beliefs.

LEGAL ISSUES

- Issues of **criminal law** deal with persons who threaten society.
- Issues of **civil law** involve violations of individual private rights.
- Civil wrongs involving individual or private property rights are called **torts**.
- Torts may be intentional, such as slander, or unintentional, such as accidental injury due to negligence.

- Substandard care or **negligence** is an example of an unintentional tort.
- Professional misconduct, incompetence, and lack of skill may be termed **malpractice**.
- **Assault** involves intended threat or harm without physical contact.
- Physically touching another person without permission, regardless of injury, characterizes **battery**.
- Failure to follow explicit policies involving the use of restraints and narcotics may result in accusations of **false imprisonment**.
- **Defamation** of someone's character may be either written (libel) or spoken (slander).
- Discussing a patient's condition in public, improper release of medical information, including x rays, is an example of **invasion of privacy**.
- Other forms of privacy invasion are exposure and unreasonable or uncalled-for treatment.
- Notifying the patient of specific procedures and the options involved in their care is known as **informed consent**.
- **Simple consent** is a term denoting that a patient has no knowledge of the procedure that will be performed and that verbal consent should be obtained.
- **Implied and expressed** consent are two types of simple consent.
- **Implied consent** refers to consent being given by another person in an emergency situation because the patient is unable to make a decision.
- **Expressed consent** is involved when a patient wants a procedure to be performed although they may not have given verbal or written approval.
- The patient should understand the nature, risks, outcomes, and alternatives of the procedure before providing consent.
- An **incident report** is required when any error in care results in harm or injury to a patient.

- Incident reports should be thorough and include the following information:
  What occurred
  The exact time of occurrence
  Where the incident took place
  Who was involved
  Who was a witness
  What the results of the incident were
  Whether any action was taken.

- Health care providers are protected from liability by **Good Samaritan laws** when helping in an emergency outside the x-ray department or hospital.

SPECIAL CONSENT TO OPERATION, POST OPERATIVE CARE, MEDICAL TREATMENT, ANESTHESIA, OR OTHER PROCEDURE

Patient:______________________ Patient No:______________

Washington State law guarantees that you have both the right and obligation to make decisions concerning your health care. Your physician can provide you with the necessary information and advice, but as a member of the health care team, you must enter into the decision making process. This form has been designed to acknowledge your acceptance of treatment recommended by your physician.

① I hereby authorize Dr.______________ and/or such associates or assistants as may be selected by said physician to treat the following condition(s) which has (have) been explained to me: (Explain the nature of the condition(s) in professional and lay language.)

____
____
____
____

② The procedures planned for treatment of my condition(s) have been explained to me by my physician. I understand them to be: (Describe procedures to be performed in professional and lay language.)

____
____
____
____
____

At:______________________
(NAME OF HOSPITAL OR MEDICAL FACILITY)

③ I recognize that, during the course of the operation, post operative care, medical treatment, anesthesia or other procedure, unforeseen conditions may necessitate additional or different procedures than those above set forth. **I therefore authorize my above named physician, and his or her assistants or designees, to perform such surgical or other procedures as are in the exercise of his, her or their professional judgment necessary and desirable.** The authority granted under this paragraph shall extend to the treatment of **all conditions** that require treatment and are not known to my physician at the time the medical or surgical procedure is commenced.

④ **I have been informed that there are significant risks** such as severe loss of blood, infection and cardiac arrest that can lead to death or permanent or partial disability, which may be attendant to the performance of any procedure. **I acknowledge that no warranty or guarantee has been made to me as to result or cure.**

IMPORTANT: HAVE PATIENT SIGN FULL OR LIMITED DISCLOSURE BOX AND SIGNATURE LINE AT BOTTOM.

Full Disclosure

I certify that my physician has informed me of the nature and character of the proposed treatment, of the anticipated results of the proposed treatment, of the possible alternative forms of treatment; and the recognized serious possible risks, complications, and the anticipated benefits involved in the proposed treatment and in the alternative forms of treatment, including non-treatment.

____
PATIENT/OTHER LEGALLY RESPONSIBLE PERSON SIGN IF APPLICABLE

Limited Disclosure

I certify that my physician has explained to me that I have the right to have clearly described to me the nature and character of the proposed treatment; the anticipated results of the proposed treatment; the alternative forms of treatment; and the recognized serious possible risks, complications, and anticipated benefits involved in the proposed treatment, and in the alternative forms of treatment, including non-treatment.

I do not wish to have these risks and facts explained to me.

____
PATIENT/OTHER LEGALLY RESPONSIBLE PERSON SIGN IF APPLICABLE

Any sections below which do not apply to the proposed treatment may be crossed out. All sections crossed out must be initialed by both physician and patient.

⑤ I consent to the administration of anesthesia by my attending physician, by an anesthesiologist, or other qualified party under the direction of a physician as may be deemed necessary. I understand that all anesthetics involve risks of complications and serious possible damage to vital organs such as the brain, heart, lung, liver and kidney and that in some cases may result in paralysis, cardiac arrest and/or brain death from both known and unknown causes.

⑥ I consent to the use of transfusion of blood and blood products as deemed necessary.

⑦ Any tissues or parts surgically removed may be disposed of by the hospital or physician in accordance with accustomed practice.

I certify this form has been fully explained to me, that I have read it or have had it read to me, that the blank spaces have been filled in, and that I understand its contents.

DATE:______________ TIME:______ A.M. P.M.

____
PATIENT/OTHER LEGALLY RESPONSIBLE PERSON SIGN

WITNESS______________________

____
RELATIONSHIP OF LEGALLY RESPONSIBLE PERSON TO PATIENT

SCH FORM NO. OR-04 (Rev. 11/87) PERFECT PRINTING

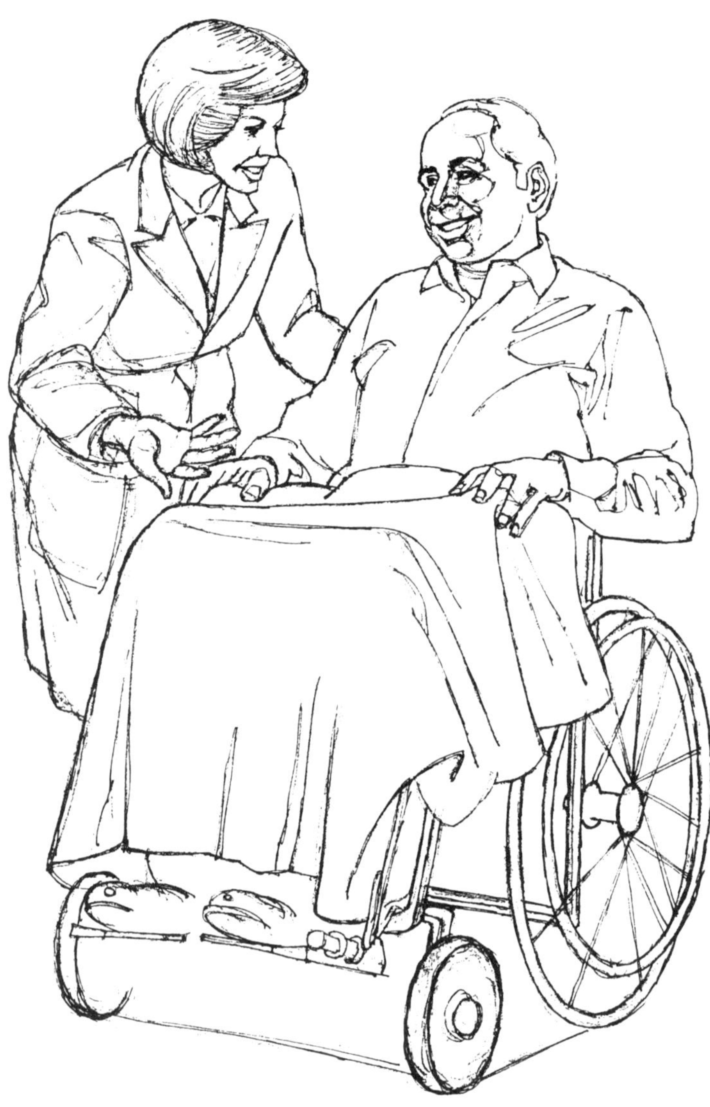

PATIENT COMMUNICATION

- **Communication** can be verbal or nonverbal.
- **Verbal** communication includes written and spoken words.
- **Nonverbal** communication includes actions, gestures, or expressions.
- **Intrapersonal** communication refers to personal communication or to communicating with oneself.
- **Interpersonal** communication is communication with others.

Special Communication Circumstances

- **Diversity** factors such as race, gender, age, educational level, and belief systems may influence the way illness is perceived and approached.
- **Sensory** alterations, such as blindness or physical impairment, may alter patient perception and require various methods of communication.
- **Chemicals** such as drugs, alcohol, or medications can alter patient cognition and require unique supervision and diversified means of communication.
- Patients with a terminal illness need effective interaction with health care professionals.
- The **five stages of grief** as noted by E. Kubler-Ross are denial, anger, bargaining, depression, and acceptance.
- It is important to note all special circumstances when communicating with patients.

Chapter 1 Review Questions

1. A civil wrong that involves individual property rights is called
   a. a tort.
   b. negligence.
   c. defamation.
   d. libel.

2. **Which of the following is based on moral responsibilities and values?**
   a. civil law
   b. criminal law
   c. ethical issues
   d. none of the above
3. **Restraining a patient without reason may constitute**
   a. defamation of character.
   b. false imprisonment.
   c. invasion of privacy.
   d. criminal law.
4. **Written defamation of a person is termed**
   a. invasion of privacy.
   b. criminal law.
   c. slander.
   d. libel.
5. **Spoken defamation of a person is called**
   a. invasion of privacy.
   b. criminal law.
   c. slander.
   d. libel.
6. **Specific responsibilities for the imaging professional can be found in**
   a. the Code of Ethics.
   b. the Principles of Conduct.
   c. the Scope of Practice.
   d. all of the above.
7. **Patients are protected by which of the following documents outlining the expectations of the patient?**
   a. Code of Ethics
   b. Principles of Conduct
   c. Scope of Practice
   d. Patient's Bill of Rights
8. **The ninth code in the ASRT Code of Ethics states that "the radiologic technologist respects confidences entrusted in the course of professional practice. . . ." Failure to practice this may result in which of the following?**
   a. defamation of character
   b. invasion of privacy
   c. malpractice
   d. negligence
9. **A process by which patients can agree to be treated or refuse to be treated based on information provided by the radiographer about specific treatment is which of the following?**
   a. implied consent
   b. informed consent
   c. simple consent
   d. inadequate consent

10. **A patient who is incapable of making the emergency decision because of mental illness can have someone else give consent for a procedure. This type of consent is termed**
    a. implied consent.
    b. informed consent.
    c. simple consent.
    d. inadequate consent.

11. **Which of the following is known as communicating with oneself?**
    a. nonverbal communication
    b. verbal communication
    c. intrapersonal communication
    d. interpersonal communication

12. **Which of the following is the first of the Kubler-Ross five stages of grief?**
    a. anger
    b. denial
    c. bargaining
    d. depression
    e. acceptance

General Patient Care

CHAPTER 2

BODY MECHANICS

- **Body mechanics** employs principles of gravity and balance to assist in the prevention of injury to the radiographer and to the patient.
- **Back injury** due to improper moving methods is the number one injury to health care workers.
- **Basic principles** involved in proper body mechanics include
  - Establishing a broad base of support for proper balance (i.e., feet spread to secure balance)
  - Correct posture that ensures the center of gravity to be in the pelvis
  - Always lifting with the leg muscles and tightening the abdominal muscles
  - Rolling or pulling heavy objects whenever possible rather than lifting or pulling.

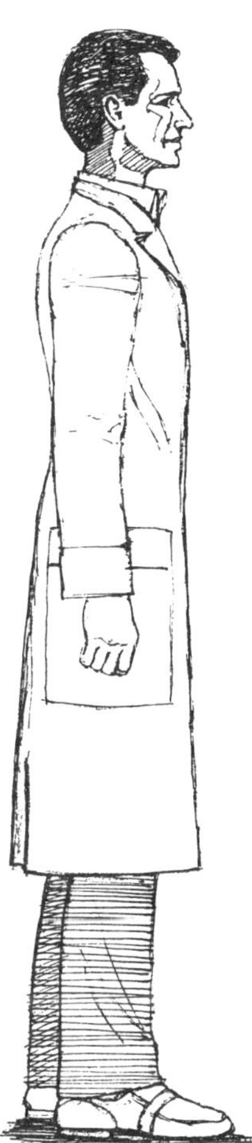

PHYSICAL STATES

- An **ambulatory** patient can walk and move with little assistance.
- Fully **immobile** patients cannot move or assist in transfer procedures.
- Paralysis from the waist down is known as **paraplegia**.
- Paralysis from the neck down is called **quadriplegia**.
- With the use of **mobilization aids** such as crutches, canes, or walkers, patients can become semimobile.

BASIC PATIENT BODY POSITIONS

- A patient is in the **supine** position when he is lying flat on his back.
- When the patient is lying flat on her abdomen, she is in the **prone** position.

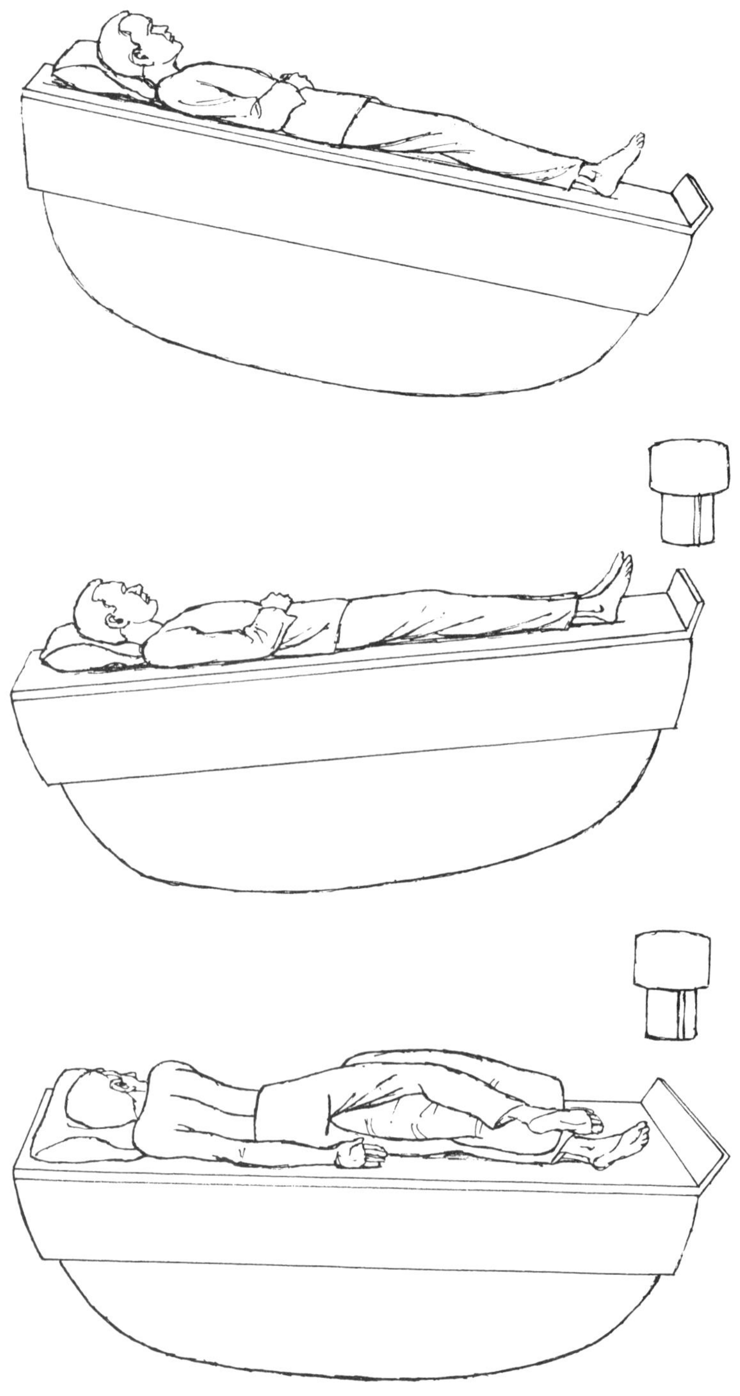

- In the **lateral** position the patient is lying on either his right or his left side.
- In **Fowler's or semi-Fowler's** position the head of the bed is elevated to place the patient in a semierect or sitting position.
- The **Trendelenburg** position is a variation of the supine position in which the patient's feet are elevated and the head is lowered.
- A patient in **Sims'** position is placed in the left lateral position with the right knee bent and drawn toward the chest. The left arm is behind and beside the patient.

TRANSFERRING PATIENTS

- **Verify** patient identity before moving a patient for any examination.
- **Evaluate** the type of transfer and any extraneous objects involved such as oxygen tubing, a urinary catheter, or intravenous (IV) tubing.
- **Assess** the situation by communicating with the patient, examining the patient for physical abnormalities, and consulting with other health care professionals when necessary.
- **Determine** the method of transfer and the patient's ability to aid in the transfer.
- **Explain** the method of transfer and provide clear directions to the patient.
- **Obtain** adequate assistance to ensure safety.

MODE OF TRANSFER

Stretcher to Table or Bed

- Moving a patient from a stretcher to a table or bed is best performed with the aid of other personnel.
- All wheels on the bed and table should be locked.
- Two people should assist from the opposite side of the table, and two should assist from the patient's side.
- The patient's condition should be assessed to evaluate the use of a slide board or draw sheets.

Wheelchair to Table or Bed

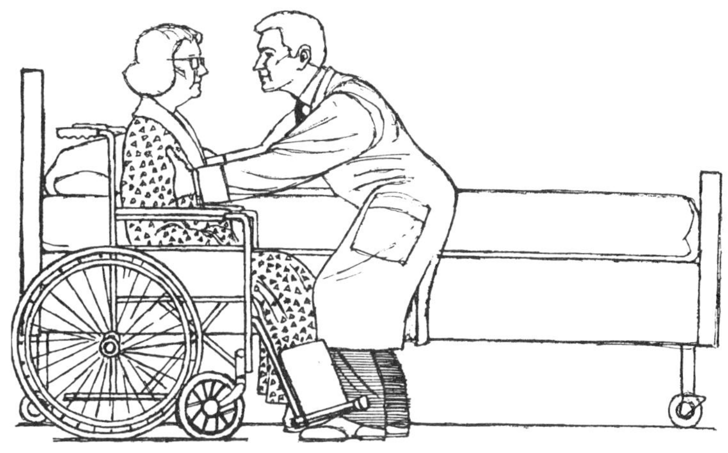

- Transfer from a wheelchair to a table or bed may require little assistance or a great amount of assistance depending on patient's condition.
- The wheelchair should be placed parallel to the table with the wheels locked before beginning the assist.
- Standing between the footrests, support and lift the patient into an upright position.
- Always squat and use the leg muscles when lifting.
- Patients with a unilateral weakness should be assisted from the affected side.

Wheelchair to Stool or Chair

- Transfers from a wheelchair to a stool or chair should be executed with patients who can assist with the move.
- A patient should never be allowed to transfer without some form of assistance.
- The technologist should assist the patient by standing directly in front of the patient in between the footrests.
- The stool or chair should be close enough to the wheelchair so that the patient can stand and either walk or pivot into the seat with assistance.
- A patient should stand upright to gain her sense of balance before being placed in the chair.

Basic Log Roll

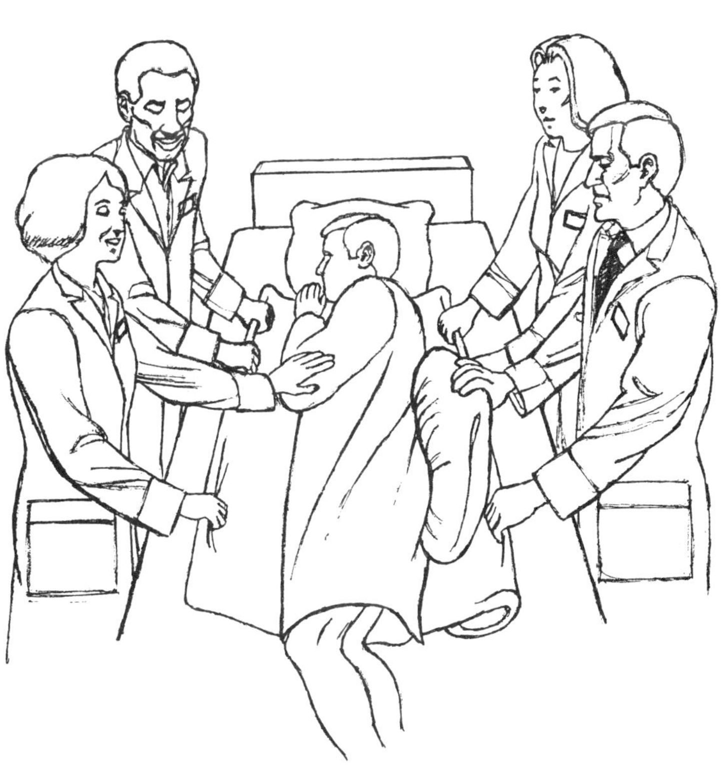

- Four to five people should assist in all log roll procedures in which the patient is under strict spine precautions.
- The patient's hands should be placed across their chest.
- Two people should be on the side on which the patient will be rolled up. One person should maintain proper head and neck alignment while one or two people maneuver the patient's torso.
- The sheet under the patient is grasped and wrapped tightly over the patient's distal side.

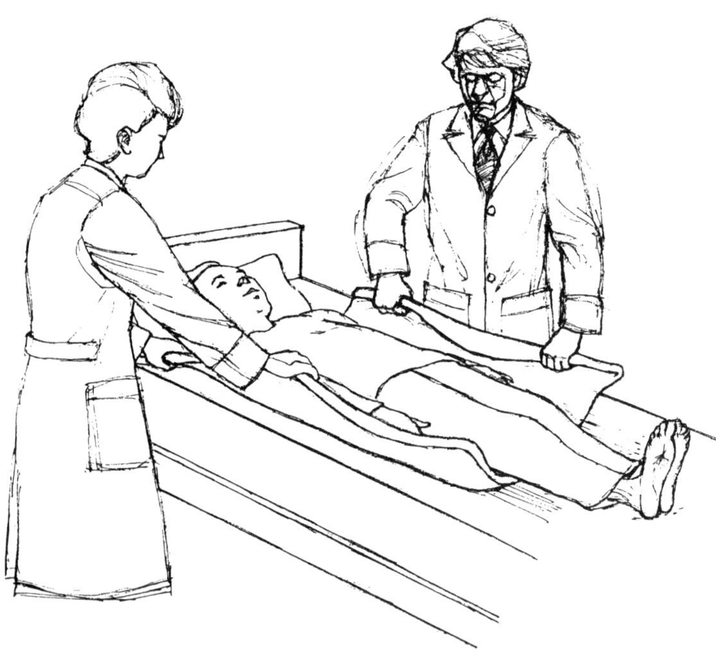

- One person should facilitate the roll to ensure that the move is performed in concert.
- Once the patient is in the desired position, reinforcement via pillows, etc., should be used.

Sheet-Assisted Transfers

- Sheet-assisted transfers require at least two people.
- A heavy sheet or blanket should be rolled longitudinally.
- One person should turn the patient onto his side, bringing him as close to the distal edge of the bed as possible.
- The person assisting should simultaneously place the sheet as close as possible to the patient's back.
- The patient should be turned back to the supine position and informed that he will be rolling over the sheet.
- The sheet should then be unrolled as the patient rolls up slightly toward the assistant.

Slide Board-Assisted Transfers

- Slide boards allow ease of movement for patients who cannot move without aid.
- Slide boards reduce the number of personnel required to assist in the move.
- A slide board should be placed under the patient's sheet.
- Using the basic log roll maneuver, slip the board as far as possible under the patient.
- Roll the patient back into the supine position and repeat the preceding step, rolling the patient in the opposite direction.
- Slide the patient onto the table using the slide board to span the gap between the gurney and the table.
- Rolling the patient in the opposite direction, remove the slide board.

HELPING THE PATIENT TO GOWN

- When removing clothing from a patient, it is important to maintain as much modesty as possible.
- When aiding a patient who has an injured extremity, remove clothing from the torso and gown the patient.
- Clothing should be slid off the legs after the top portion of the patient is covered with a gown.
- Patients with total paralysis, or those unable to cooperate, should first be covered with a sheet before removing their clothing.
- It is important to obtain assistance whenever gowning a patient who is entirely unable to help with the procedure.
- Clothing should be removed from the patient's unaffected side first.
- When gowning a patient, first place the arm of the affected side into the gown.
- Always maintain patient modesty while removing clothing by using a sheet or blanket cover.
- It may be necessary to log-roll the patient in order to remove all articles of clothing.

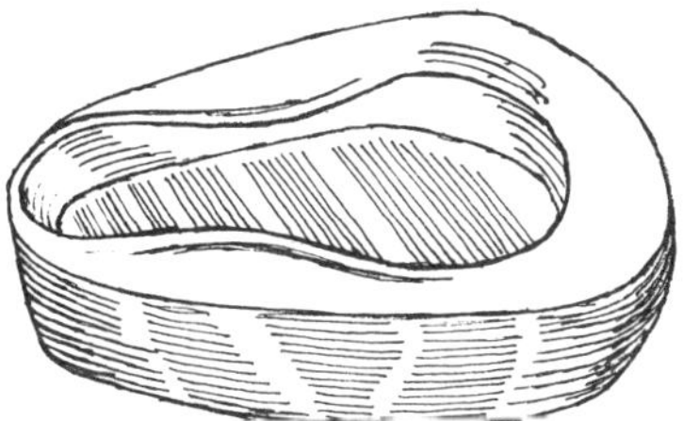

ELIMINATION NEEDS

- Patients who cannot walk require the use of a urinal or a bedpan.
- Always wear gloves when assisting a patient with elimination needs.
- If the patient cannot lift her hips for placement or removal of the bedpan, lay her flat, have her roll away from you, and gently place or remove the bedpan from under the pelvis.

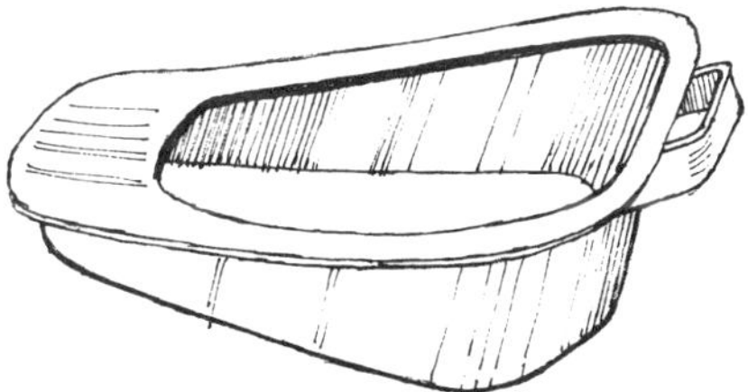

- Always check the patient's chart to observe whether urine output is being measured.
- Fracture bedpans are smaller, more shallow at one end, and easier to place.
- With male patients, urinals should be used by placing the penis in the urinal.
- Urine or fecal material should be disposed of immediately and properly.
- Gloves should be discarded and hands washed.

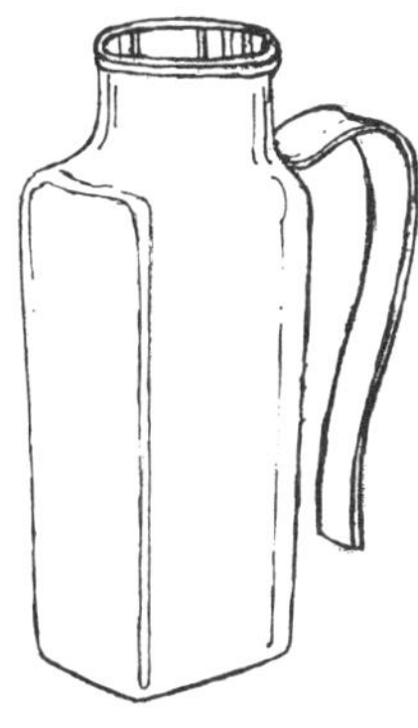

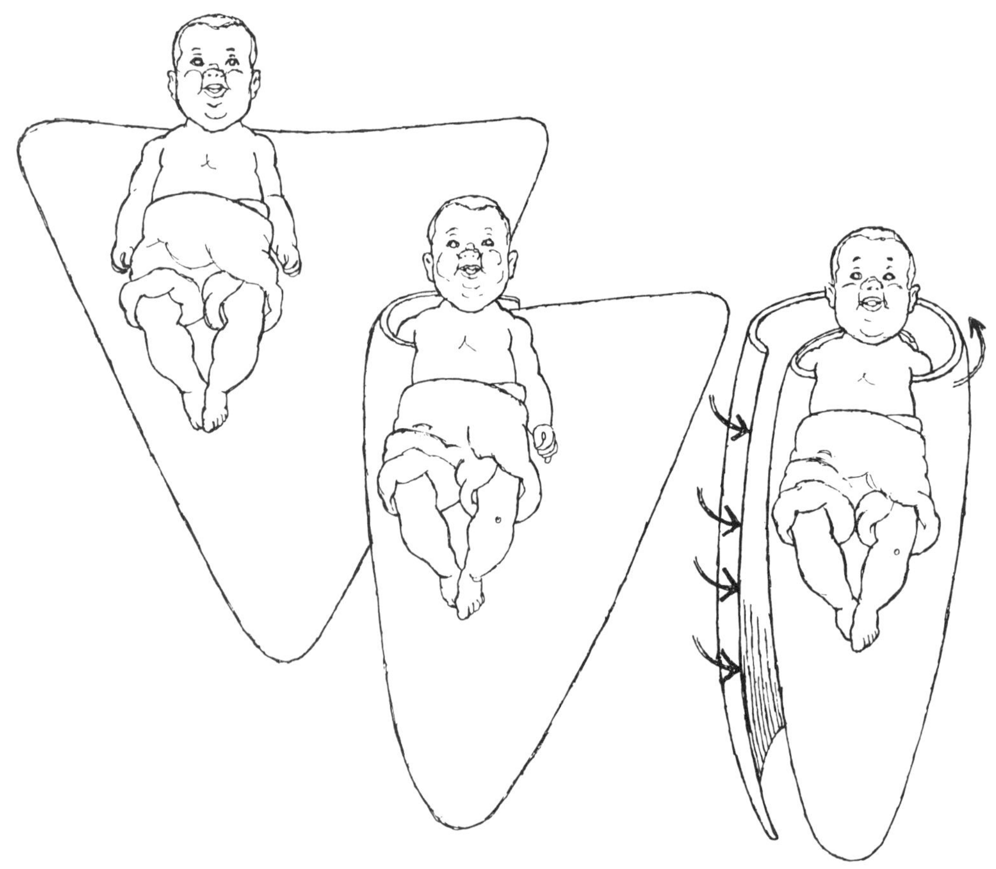

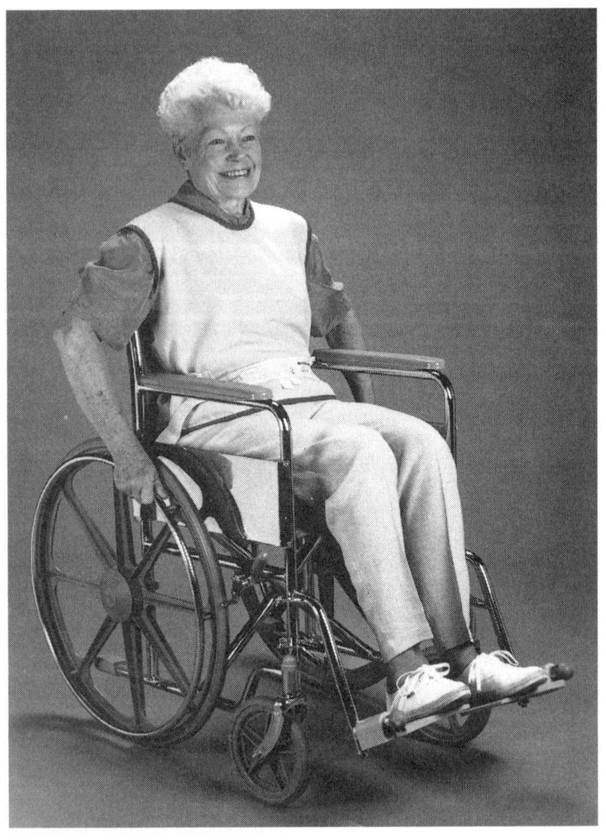

METHODS FOR RESTRAINING A PATIENT

- Imaging professionals should not hold patients during radiation exposure in order to restrain them in a specific position.
- Methods of restraint should be used only when no other safe measures to accomplish the examination are possible.
- A Pig-O-Stat, papoose board, or sheet may be used to form a mummy restraint for infants and toddlers.
- Ankle, limb, or four-point restraints are usually used with a patient who is on a gurney or bed.
- Wrist restraints can be used with either a gurney or a wheelchair.
- A vest or waist restraint allows examination safety and minor movement of the patient.
- A cervical collar allows restricted movement of the spine.

Legality of Restraint

- Restraints should be used only for patients who must be maintained in a particular position, to control a site for IV or catheter injection, or to preserve the safety of an impaired patient.
- Chart documentation is required when it is necessary for a patient to be restrained.
- Patients should be placed in restraints for extended periods only with the written order of a physician.
- All restrained patients should be carefully monitored.
- Padded restraints should be used.
- Security personnel should assist in restraining all combative patients.
- The minimum amount of time, with respect for safety, should be spent in restraints.

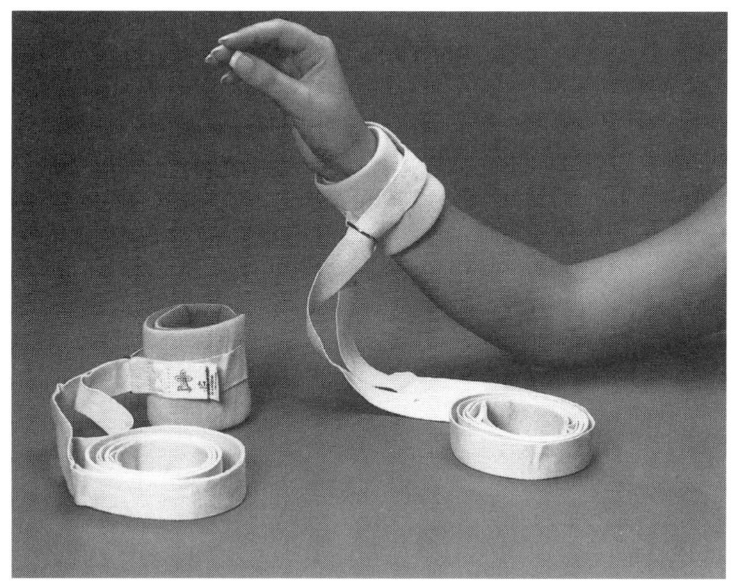

Chapter 2 Review Questions

1. **When transferring patients, the radiographer should be sure that**
   a. the wheels are locked on the wheelchair, bed, or gurney.
   b. communication has ensured that the patient understands the procedure.
   c. necessary personnel are employed to help assist in the move.
   d. all of the above are true.

2. **When using a slide board to move an immobile patient, it is best to use which of the following methods?**
   a. Push the patient onto the slide board.
   b. Roll the patient onto the slide board.
   c. Using a draw sheet and other personnel to assist, pull the patient onto the slide board.
   d. Ask the patient to help move himself onto the slide board.

3. **What is the primary determinant to be considered when evaluating the method of transfer?**
   a. type of examination
   b. strength of the professional moving the patient
   c. gender of the patient
   d. all of the above

4. **Ambulatory means which of the following?**
   a. The patient required the use of a stretcher.
   b. The patient requires the use of a wheelchair.
   c. The patient must stay in bed.
   d. The patient is able to walk.

5. **A patient lying flat on her back is said to be in**
   a. the supine position.
   b. the Trendelenburg position.
   c. Sims' position.
   d. Fowler's position.

6. **When undressing a patient with an injury to the upper torso, one should**
   a. remove clothing from the injured or affected side first.
   b. remove clothing from the uninjured or unaffected side first.
   c. pay no attention to how the clothing is removed.
   d. put the hospital gown on over the patient's clothing.

7. **Which of the following types of patients require assistance from other personnel in order to facilitate a move?**
   a. ambulatory
   b. mobile
   c. immobile
   d. all of the above

8. **In order to reduce body strain, when moving patients it is best to**
   a. pull rather than push them.
   b. push rather than pull them.
   c. push or pull them, whichever can complete the move.
   d. do none of the above.

9. **Which of the following is not a principle of body mechanics?**
   a. feet spread to secure balance
   b. correct posture
   c. knees locked and leg muscles tightened
   d. pull whenever possible

10. **Which mode of movement is best when radiographing patients with spinal injuries?**
    a. a two-person lift using a draw sheet
    b. a five-person log roll with slide board assistance
    c. moving the shoulders onto the table and then following with the feet
    d. asking the patient if they can assist in the move

11. **Before moving a patient for examination, which of the following is most important?**
    a. verifying the patient's identity
    b. assessing the patient's condition
    c. employing adequate assistance
    d. explaining the examination to the patient

12. **Which of the following should be done when assisting a patient with elimination needs?**
    a. Assist with placement of the urinal or bedpan.
    b. Check the patient's chart to observe if urine output is being measured.
    c. Dispose of all waste immediately if measurements are not required.
    d. All of the above.

13. **Which type of restraint is best used with a patient in a wheelchair?**
    a. vest restraint
    b. ankle restraints
    c. wrist restraints
    d. any method of restraint
14. **Who has the authority to restrain a patient?**
    a. the imaging professional conducting the examination
    b. the patient's nurse
    c. the patient's physician
    d. all of the above
15. **Which of the following is a reason to restrain a patient?**
    a. to maintain a specific position
    b. to guard a patient's safety
    c. to temporarily immobilize an intravenous site
    d. all of the above

CHAPTER 3

Vital Signs

TEMPERATURE

- **Three sites** commonly used for taking body temperature are the mouth, axilla, and rectum.
- **Body temperature** usually causes physiological changes when it fluctuates 2 to 3 degrees.
- **Fluctuations** may be caused by the following factors:
  Time of day
  Environment and quantity of exercise
  Age
  Hormone levels
  Emotions
  Disease process.
- Normal **oral temperature** ranges from 97 to 99°F or 36 to 37.5°C.
- Normal **axillary temperature** ranges from 96.5 to 98.5°F or 35.5 to 37°C.
- Normal **rectal temperature** values range from 97.5 to 99.5°F or 36.5 to 38°C.
- A clinical **glass thermometer** is a glass bulb containing mercury.
- Clinical glass thermometers should be shaken to move the mercury below the normal level.
- Temperature is measured using an **oral glass thermometer** when the mercury in the bulb expands due to heating.
- Oral glass thermometers can measure both axillary and oral temperatures.
- A **rectal glass thermometer** is distinguished by its red-tipped end and measures temperature using the same principle as an oral thermometer.
- The **scale** used on clinical thermometers is located on the stem and ranges from 95°F (35°C) to 110°F (43.3°C).

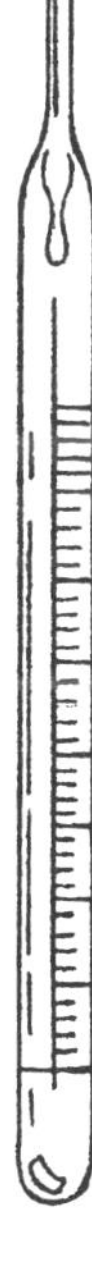

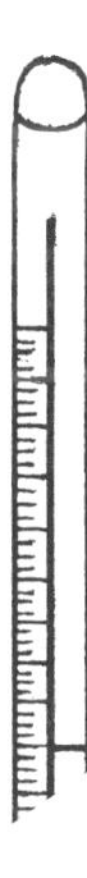

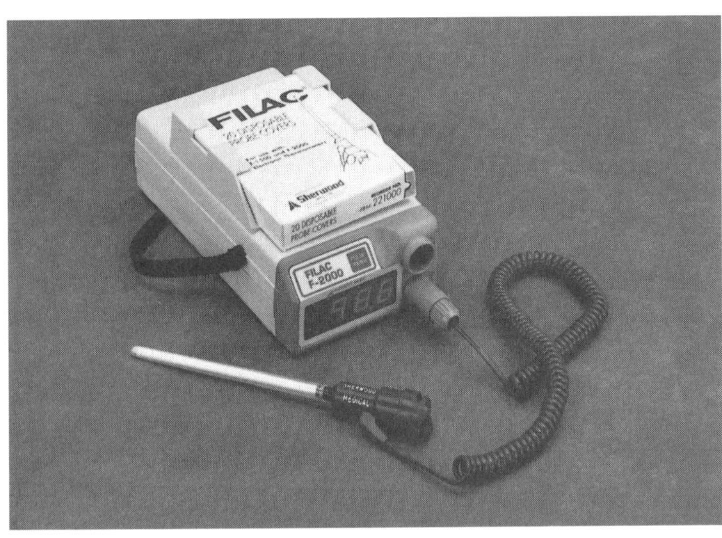

- All temperatures measured with clinical glass thermometers should be recorded as ending in **even tenths**, e.g., 99.2°F.
- **Electronic oral thermometers** are portable, are battery-operated, and can usually measure a temperature in seconds.
- The temperature on an electronic thermometer is displayed digitally in either odd or even tenths of a degree.
- **Tympanic thermometers** use an auditory canal probe and can be adjusted to display core, oral, or rectal temperature in either Fahrenheit or Celsius.
- **Disposable thermometers** consist of temperature-sensitive tapes or ready-strip thermometers.

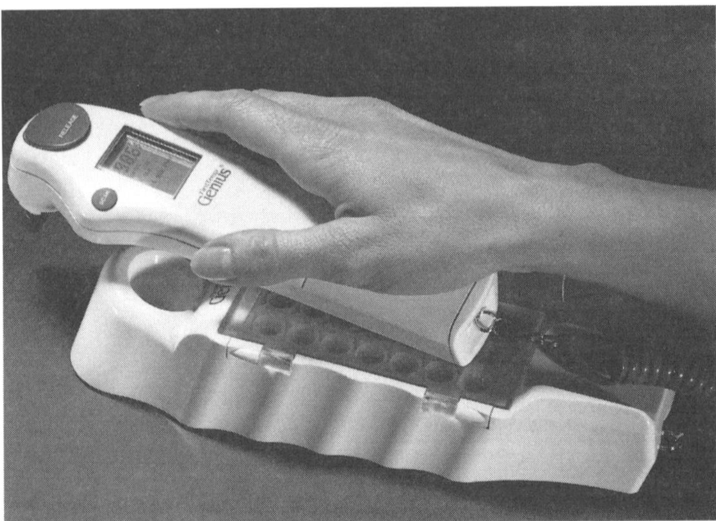

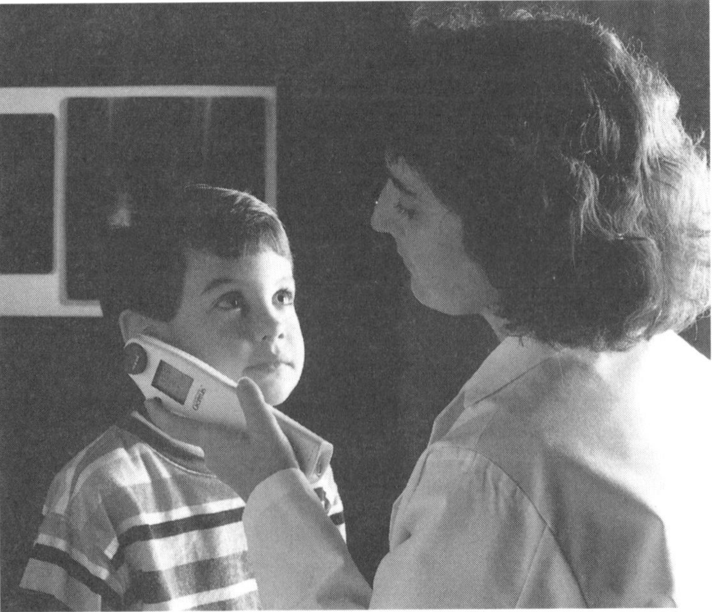

MEASURING PULSE

- Contraction of the walls of the heart to push blood into the arteries is termed and counted as a patient's **pulse**.
- The **sites** where one can determine a patient's pulse are the following:
  Temporal (anterior to the superior portion of the ear)
  Carotid (at anterior portion of neck)
  Apical (at the peak of the heart)
  Radial (at the base of the thumb)
  Femoral (in the medial groin region)
  Popliteal (at the posterior aspect of the knee)
  Pedal (either on the medial ankle or on the dorsal surface of the foot).
- The **radial artery** is the most common site for measuring pulse rate.
- The **radial pulse** is measured using the first two fingers placed on the lateral side of the wrist at the base of the thumb.

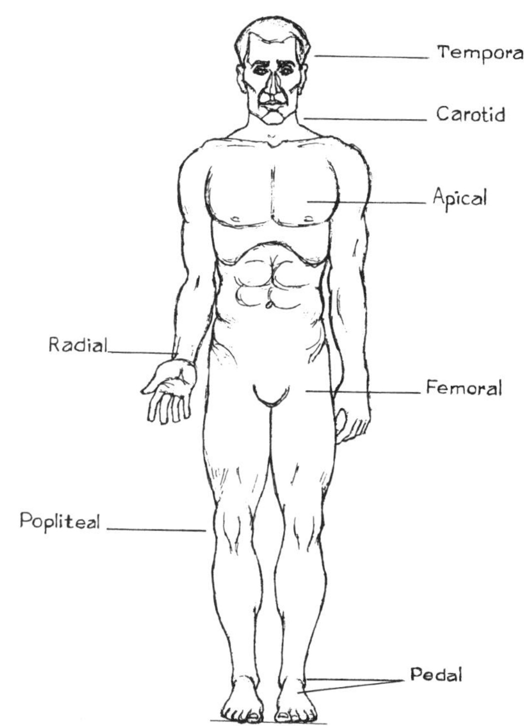

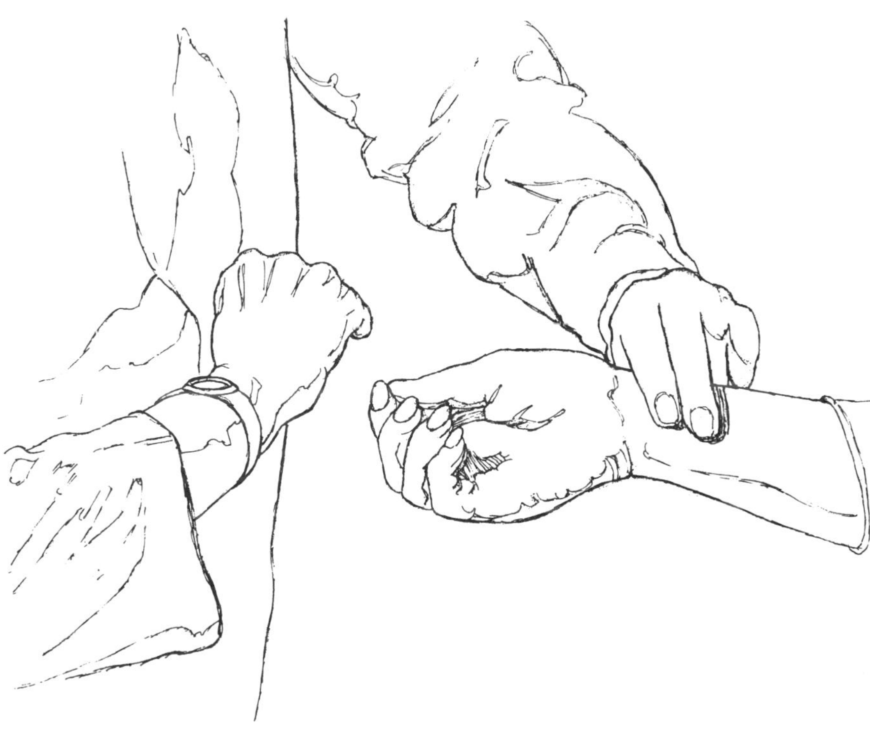

- The **apical pulse** it the most accurate measurement of a patient's pulse rate.
- The **average adult** pulse rate ranges from 70 to 100 beats per minute (BPM).
- The **average infant** pulse rate ranges from 100 to 180 BPM.

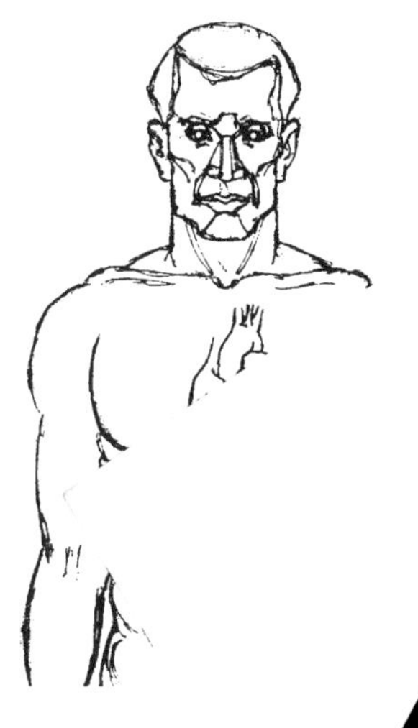

- The **average child** pulse rate ranges from 95 to 110 BPM.
- The **average adult athlete** pulse rate ranges from 45 to 60 BPM.
- **Tachycardia** (accelerated)refers to a pulse rate of more than 100 BPM minute in the average adult.
- **Bradycardia** (sluggish) is characterized by a pulse rate of less than 60 beats per minute in the average adult.
- **Factors** that may affect pulse rates are the following:
  Age, build, and body size
  Blood pressure
  Emotions
  Drugs
  Exercise
  Increased body temperature
  Pain.
- **Characteristics** to note when calculating a pulse are rate, rhythm, and volume.

RESPIRATION

- **Respiration** is the process by which the body exchanges oxygen and carbon dioxide.
- **External respiration** refers to the delivery of oxygen to the lungs.
- **Internal respiration** refers to the delivery of oxygen to and exchange of carbon dioxide with the cells.

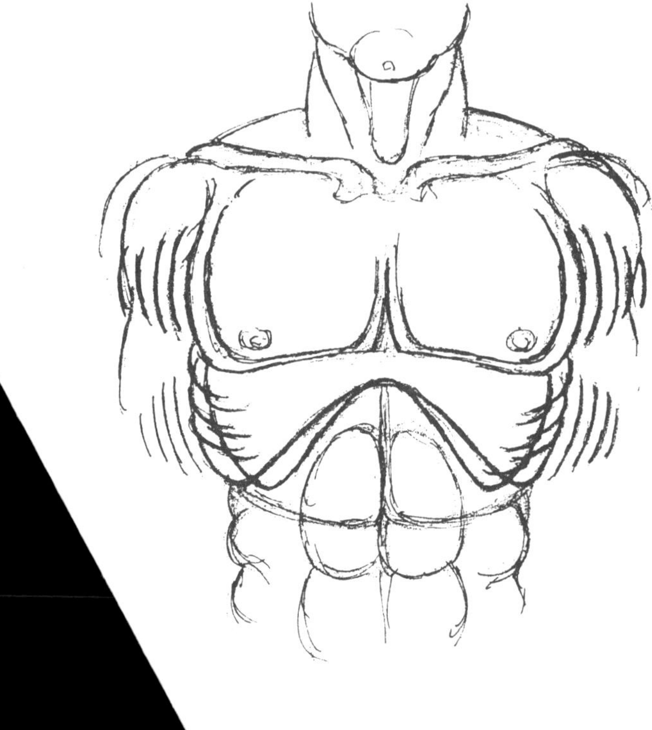

- During **inhalation** the chest expands, the diaphragm descends, and the ribs expand while moving superiorly.
- During **exhalation** the chest relaxes, the diaphragm rises, and the ribs contract while moving inferiorly.
- The rate of respiration for a **normal adult** is 14 to 20 respirations per minute.
- The rate of respiration for a **youth** is 16 to 20 respirations per minute.
- The rate of respiration for a **child** is 20 to 30 respirations per minute.
- The rate of respiration for an **infant** is 35 or more respirations per minute.

- The relative number of respirations may be influenced by the following:
  - Emotions
  - Pain
  - Activity and age
  - Drugs and disease
  - Temperature.
- The **ratio** of respiration to heartbeats is approximately 1 to 4.
- Respirations should be observed for differences in pattern, effort, and rate.
- **Dyspnea** is difficult or strained breathing.
- **Tachypnea** is increased or rapid respiration.
- Decreased oxygen in the blood, or **hypoxia**, can be caused by slow or shallow breathing patterns.
- Respirations in which dyspnea is followed by apnea are termed **Cheyne-Stokes respirations.**
- **Hyperventilation** occurs when carbon dioxide levels are low. Respirations have increased rate and depth.

BLOOD PRESSURE

- **Blood pressure** (**BP**) is a product of the following:
  - Intensity of the contraction of the heart ventricle
  - Amount of blood being pumped out of the heart
  - Resistance of blood vessels to blood flow.
- The **systolic pressure** denotes the force of ventricular contraction.
- The **diastolic pressure** denotes the lowest pressure of the ventricle between heartbeats.
- Blood pressure is **written** with the systolic pressure over the diastolic pressure.
- A **sphygmomanometer** and a **stethoscope** are the instruments used to measure blood pressure.
- Blood pressure is measured in **millimeters of mercury** which is charted as mm Hg.

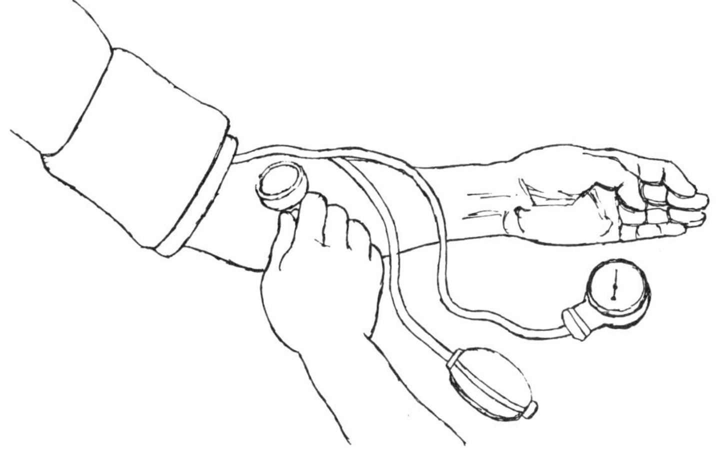

Measuring Blood Pressure

- BP can be measured in the sitting, standing, or lying position.

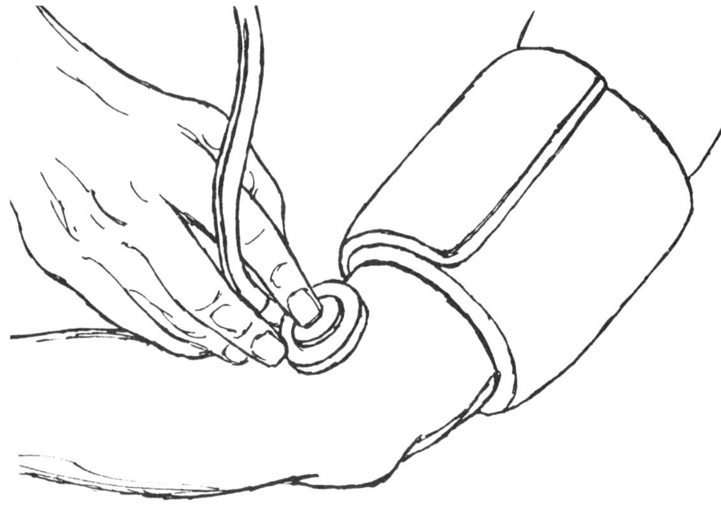

- Measurements are usually taken in the **brachial artery** at the distal humerus.
- The **cuff** of the sphygmomanometer should be positioned around the bare arm.
- The **bell** of the stethoscope should be placed directly over the artery.
- With the **pressure screw** tightened, the bulb should be pumped until the gauge reads at least 180 mm Hg.
- The pressure screw should then be slowly loosened, allowing the needle of the gauge to drop no more than 2 mm Hg per second.
- **Systolic pressure** is noted when the pulse is first heard.
- **Diastolic pressure** is noted when the rhythm is at its softest.

  Factors that affect blood pressure may be the following:
  - Age and gender
  - Body build
  - Activity
  - Body stance or position
  - Emotions
  - Pathology or disease
  - Hemorrhage.
- **Hypertension** is the term used to describe elevated blood pressure.
- **Hypotension** denotes low blood presure.
- **Normal BP values** for children, adolescents, and adults are

Age Group	Systolic	Diastolic
Children (8–11)	105 (±15)	60 (±10)
Adolescents	85–130	45–85
Adults	90–140	60–90

- Measurements for **infants and small children** should be taken in series because of the range of acceptable values.
- **Korotkoff sounds** may be noted when measuring blood pressure and may have the following characteristics:
  - Knocking occurring with heartbeat
  - Muffling during diastolic pressure
  - Silence during diastolic pressure
  - Swishing while the cuff is collapsing
  - Tapping during systolic pressure.

Chapter 3 Review Questions

1. **Which of the following is the normal rectal temperature range?**
   a. 97° to 99°F
   b. 96.5° to 98.5°F
   c. 97.5° to 99.5°F
   d. 98.5° to 100°F

2. **Which of the following could cause a fluctuation in body temperature?**
   a. exercise
   b. time of day
   c. hormones
   d. all of the above

3. **The oral thermometer measures temperature at which of the following sites?**

   I. oral   II. axillary   III. rectal

   a. only I
   b. only I and II
   c. only I and III
   d. all of the above

4. **Physiologic changes in the body may occur if body temperature fluctuates more than**
   a. 0.5°F.
   b. 1.0°F.
   c. 2.0 to 3.0°F.
   d. 4.0 to 5.0°F.

5. **Methods of measuring temperature include all of the following devices except**
   a. a glass mercury-filled thermometer.
   b. a tympanic thermometer.
   c. an electronic thermometer.
   d. an oximeter thermometer.

6. **Which of the following is the most common site for measuring a patient's pulse?**
   a. carotid artery
   b. apical artery
   c. temporal artery
   d. radial artery

7. **Which of the following is the site that records the most accurate pulse rate?**
   a. carotid artery
   b. apical artery
   c. temporal artery
   d. radial artery

8. **Which of the following ranges reflects an average pulse rate for a child?**
   a. 45 to 60 BPM
   b. 70 to 100 BPM
   c. 95 to 110 BPM
   d. 100 to 180 BPM

9. **When obtaining a pulse rate, which of the following characteristics should be noted?**
    a. rate
    b. rhythm
    c. volume
    d. all of the above

10. **The term used to describe difficulty in breathing is**
    a. tachycardia.
    b. dyspnea.
    c. tachypnea.
    d. brachypnea.

11. **Which of the following terms denotes the delivery of oxygen to the lungs?**
    a. respiration
    b. internal respiration
    c. external respiration
    d. Cheyne-stokes respiration

12. **The average rate of respiration for an adult is usually**
    a. 14 to 20 respirations per minute.
    b. 20 to 25 respirations per minute.
    c. 25 to 30 respirations per minute.
    d. 35+ respirations per minute.

13. **The number of heartbeat(s) per respiration is approximately**
    a. one.
    b. two.
    c. three.
    d. four.

14. **Which of the following is used to calculate blood pressure?**
    I. intensity of ventricular contraction
    II. amount of blood being pumped from the heart
    III. resistance of the vessels to the flow

    a. I and II
    b. I and III
    c. II and III
    d. I, II, and III

15. **The lowest pressure of the ventricle between each heartbeat is called the**
    a. systolic pressure.
    b. diastolic pressure.
    c. ventricular pressure.
    d. arterial pressure.

16. **When charting blood pressure, the ______ is written over the ______.**
    a. arterial
    b. systolic
    c. diastolic
    d. ventricular

17. **Which of the following terms is used to describe elevated blood pressure?**
    a. hypertension
    b. hypotension
    c. systolic tension
    d. distention

18. **An adult normal blood pressure value could be which of the following?**
    a. 60 mm Hg, 100 mm Hg
    b. 100 mm Hg, 60 mm Hg
    c. 140 mm Hg, 100 mm Hg
    d. 100 mm Hg, 100 mm Hg

Procedures for Infection Control

CHAPTER 4

- **Infection** is defined as an invasion and growth of microorganisms that cause harm to cells and tissues.
- **Microorganisms** are microscopic living organisms that cannot move about on their own.
- **Examples** of microorganisms include fungi, bacteria, yeast, viruses, and molds.
- The most common manner of **movement** for microorganisms is via air currents.
- Anything exposed to air is exposed to microorganisms.
- Since microorganisms have weight, they can be acted on by gravity and usually **settle on surfaces**.
- The **greatest accumulation** of microorganisms is on the floor.
- Growth of microorganisms is encouraged by a warm, dark, moist environment.
- **Nutrients**, such as human and animal, are required in order for microorganisms to live.

PATHOGENIC MICROORGANISMS

- **Pathogenic** is a term used to denote anything that causes infection.
- **Pathogens** are disease-causing microorganisms.
- Only a small percentage of the many microorganisms known are believed to be pathogens.
- **Illness** due to pathogens depends on factors that include
  - Environmental state
  - Number and strength of the invading pathogens
  - Ability of the host to resist invasion.

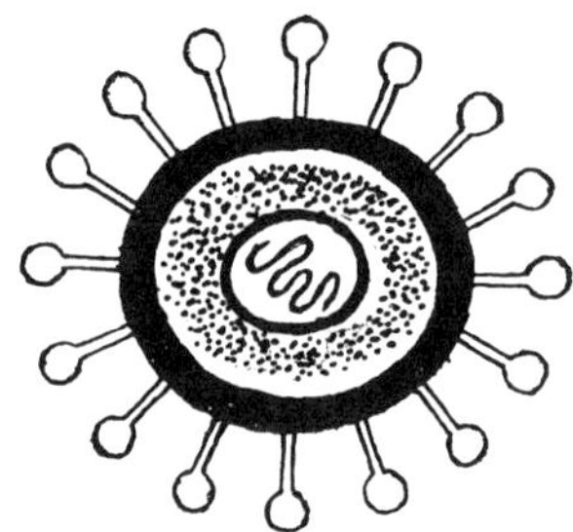

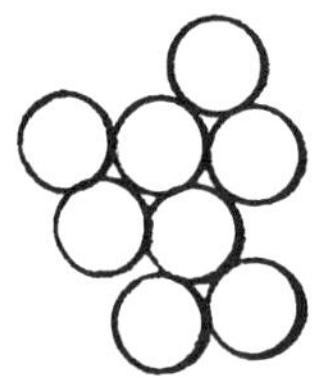

Main Types of Pathogens

- The **four main types** of pathogens are bacteria, fungi, viruses, and parasites.
- **Bacteria** are one-celled microorganisms which have both DNA and RNA.
- **Classification of bacteria** is determined based on the shape of the bacteria, their dividing characteristics, or their reaction to laboratory staining tests.
- **Shape** classifications are usually spherical, oblong, or spiral.
- **Dividing characteristics** may include pairs, chains, or bunches.
- Laboratory **testing** involves the ability of bacteria to resist staining a slide in laboratory procedures.
- In order to protect themselves, bacteria may form spores.
- A **spore** is a protective coating that forms around the nucleus of the bacteria.
- Bacteria are adaptable to various situations, which has made them resistant to may types of drugs.
- **Fungi** exist as either yeasts or molds.
- **Yeasts** are one-celled organisms.
- **Molds** are multicelled pathogenic organisms.
- **Viruses** are the smallest type of microorganism known to produce disease.
- Unlike that of bacteria, the material of a virus can be either DNA or RNA but never both.
- Viruses must invade the cell of a host in order to live.
- The outer coating, or **capsid**, of a virus is the mechanism of transport to the pathogen.
- A virus invades only a specific type of cell.
- **Multiplication** of the virus may rely on the health of the host.
- Viruses may have **dormant stages**.
- **Factors** such as stress and poor health may allow a virus to manifest, multiply, and cause acute infection.

- **Parasitic infection agents** include protozoa and helminths.
- **Protozoa** are complex one-celled microorganisms.
- Protozoa have the ability to form into **cysts** and protect themselves.
- Usually protozoa cause abnormalities in the gastrointestinal (GI), genitourinary (GU), and hematopoietic systems.
- **Helminths** are worms that can be either round (aschelminths) or flat (platyhelminths).
- Helminths have the ability to survive undetected for long periods of time.
- These parasites are usually found in the GI tract.
- Positive diagnosis requires an examination of the eggs.

STAGES OF INFECTION

- There are **four basic stages** of infection: latent period, incubation period, disease period, and convalescent period.

Stages of Infection

Latent Period →	Incubation Period →	Disease Period →	Convalescent Period
Host is entered. Host feels no symptoms.	Microorganism reproduces. Infection begins.	Symptoms are manifested. Host is communicable.	Organism may become latent. Disease may still be communicable. Symptoms may cease.

- During the **latent period** the pathogen enters the host and lies dormant.
- The host usually feels no symptoms during the latent period.
- The **incubation period** is the period during which the microorganism starts to reproduce and infection begins.
- Once infection commences, the disease process also starts.

- During the **disease period**, the host notices symptoms of the disease and is most communicable.
- With the onset of **convalescence**, the microorganism may enter a latent period in which no symptoms are exhibited.
- Some diseases may still be communicable during convalescence.

NOSOCOMIAL INFECTIONS

- Infections that are contracted within the health care environment are termed **nosocomial infections**.
- **Factors** influencing the possibility of contracting a nosocomial infection include a patient's health, environment, and drug therapy.
- Patients in the hospital are usually in poor health, which increases the risk of nosocomial infections.
- The health care facility is an environment laden with infectious microbes as a result of air contamination and because of visitors, patients, or equipment that may harbor microorganisms.
- Drug therapy designed to treat diseases such as cancer or inhibit the rejection of organ transplant suppresses the patient's immune system and makes him or her **susceptible** to pathogens.

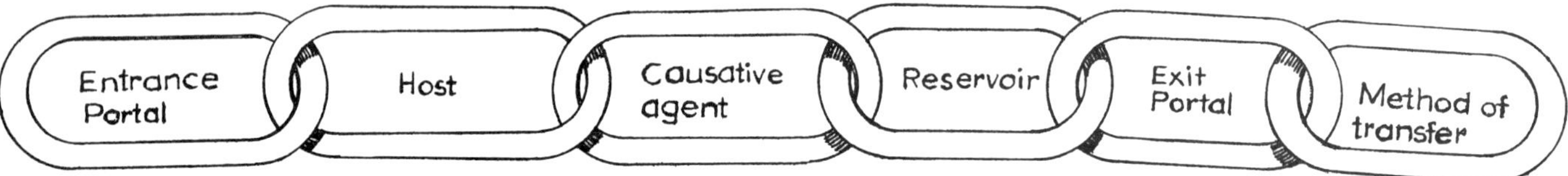

CHAIN OF INFECTION

- The **chain of infection** is a series of events that must be broken in order to prevent the spread of infection.
- The requirements necessary for the transmission of infections include
  - An infectious medium
  - A life-sustaining reservoir
  - A course by which to exit the reservoir
  - A method for conveying infection
  - A course by which to enter a new organism
  - An unprotected host.

- **Infectious media** include any of the pathogenic microorganisms mentioned previously.
- **Reservoirs** that can sustain the life of these organisms include any environment that supports the existence of the specific pathogen.
- Normal **channels** through which pathogens exit are areas that contain blood or body fluid secretions.
- Areas of injury are also points of exit for microorganisms.
- There are four basic modes of **conveying infection:** contact, vehicle, air, and vector.
- **Spread** of infection by contact may be due to direct, indirect, or droplet contact.
- **Direct contact** includes transfer by the actual touch of the infected host.
- Direct contact is the most common method of transporting infection.
- Examples of direct contact include pathogens being transfered via a contaminated x-ray cassette.
- **Indirect contact** is transfer via an object previously contaminated by the infected host.
- An example of indirect contact may be touching cassettes contaminated by the host and then touching another patient.
- Fomites are involved in the spread of infection through indirect contact.
- A **fomite** is any substance that may adhere to or aid in the transmission of infectious material.
- **Droplet contact** is accomplished via the spray or mist expelled from the mouth or nose during a cough or sneeze.
- **Vehicle contact** involves the spread of disease that has been deposited in a medium which then spreads the infection.
- Methods of vehicular transmission include food, water, blood, or drugs that have been contaminated.

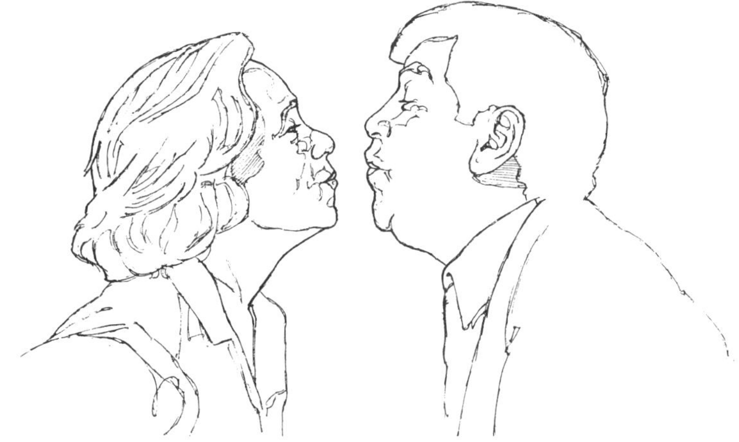

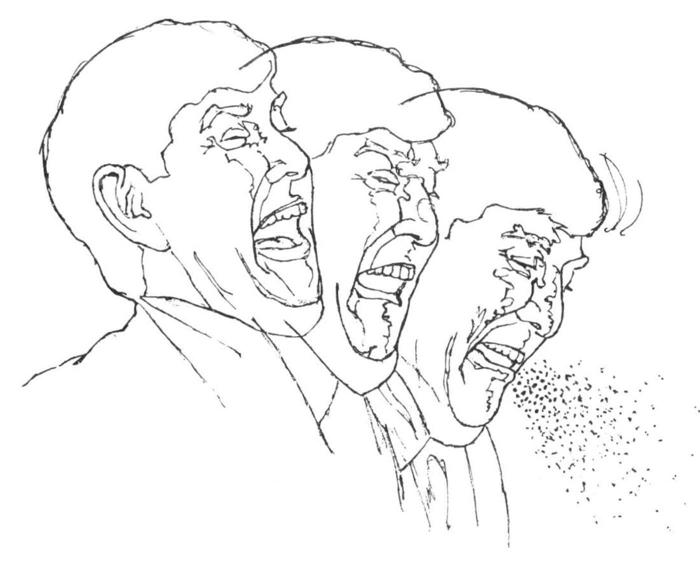

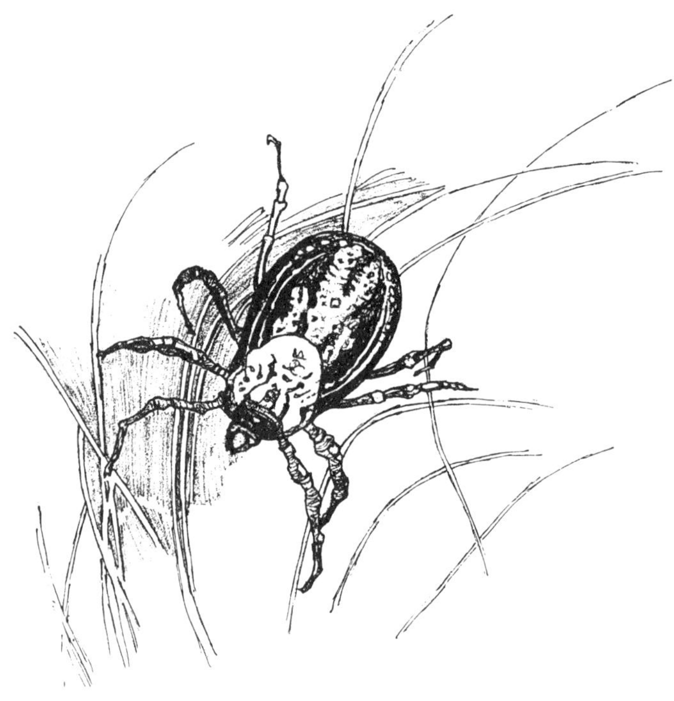

- Air acts to convey infections by spreading evaporated droplet pathogens.
- Evaporated droplets settle in dust and may then be inhaled by an unprotected host.
- **Vector infections** are actualized with the assistance of another organism such as a tick or mosquito.
- An example of a vector spreading infection is the tick and the spread of Lyme disease.
- The **course** by which the pathogen enters a new organism may be through injection, a break in the skin, ingestion, or across a mucous membrane.
- A new host is usually susceptible because of poor nourishment, poor hygiene, poor skin and wound care, and a history of chronic afflictions.
- In order to **prevent** the spread of pathogens, at least one link in the chain of infection must be broken.
- Breaking the chain of infection may be accomplished through the body's natural defense or through implementation of universal precautions.
- **The foremost way to break the chain of infection within the health care environment is through proper hand washing.**

BODILY DEFENSE AGAINST PATHOGENS

- Basic forms of **natural defense** include the skin, hair, mucous membranes, and the hematopoietic system.
- The skin, hair, muscosa, and bloodstream are nonspecific as to which pathogens they react to.
- Normally a reaction is produced by these defenses despite the type of invading bacteria.
- White blood cells or phagocytes act to ingest bacteria that may reach the bloodstream.
- **Antigens** are alien substances that invade the body.

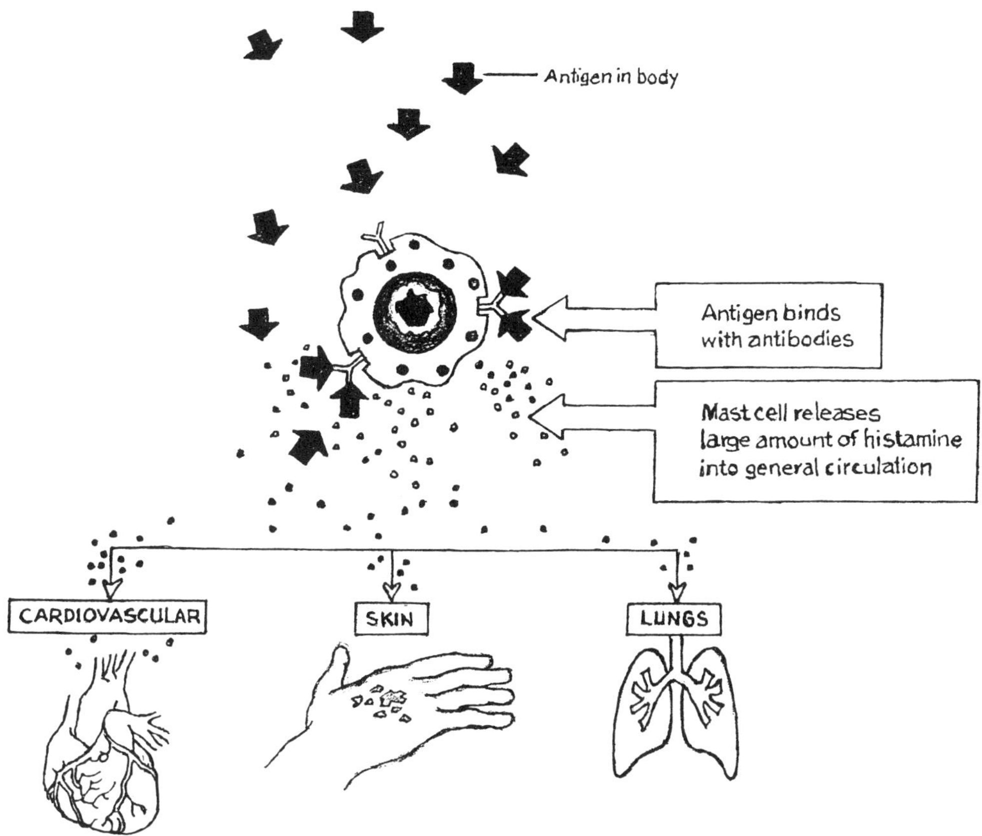

- The immune system responds to specific invaders by forming antibodies.
- **Antibodies** are protein substances that form the basis of immunity.
- Immunity can be either natural or acquired.
- A person can be born with natural immunity which is inherited and considered permanent.
- **Natural immunity** is the reason why animals may be susceptible to a specific pathogen that does not affect humans.
- **Acquired immunity** may be obtained by active or passive means.
- **Active acquired immunity** necessitates that a person meet any of the following criteria:
  - Contraction of the disease previously
  - Prior, sometimes mild infection with the disease
  - Vaccination.
- **Passive acquired immunity** requires that a person be injected with antibodies from the blood of another person or animal.

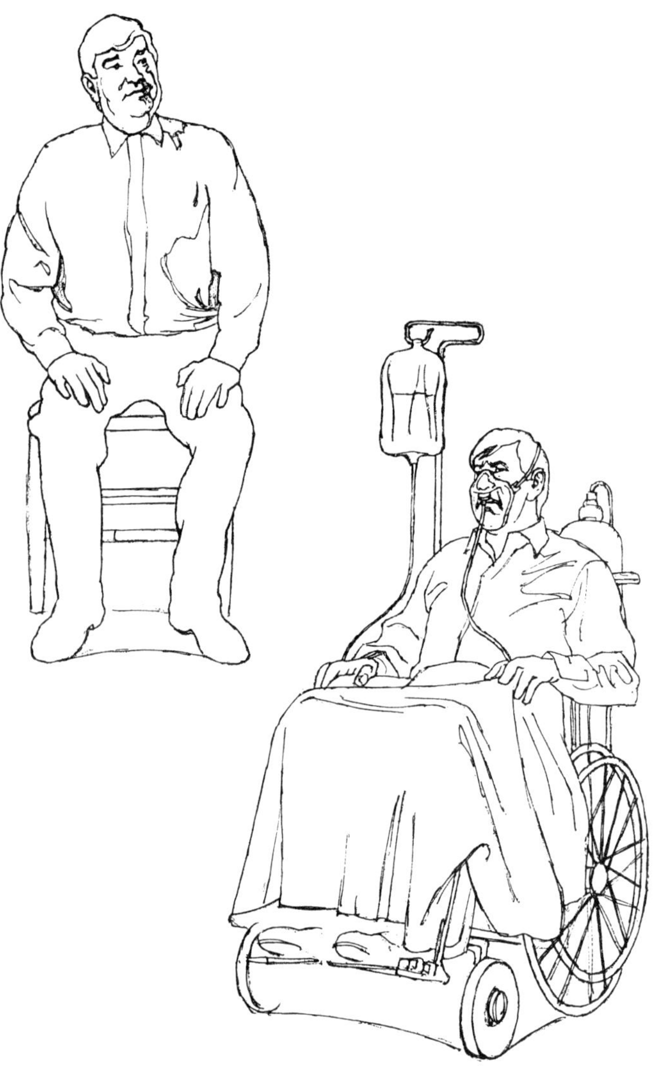

- Passive acquired immunity lasts for a short duration because it does not stimulate the person receiving antibodies to produce his own.

Resistance to Pathogens

- The **extent** of injury caused by a microorganism may be due either to the host's ability to resist or to the pathogen's ability to injure.
- **Resistance** may be **affected** by any of the following factors:
  - A person's age
  - A person's state of health
  - The presence of a disease process
  - The blood supply
  - The location of the infection
  - Anxiety or stress
  - Previously acquired antibodies.
- The ability of human beings to resist pathogens varies from individual to individual.
- Exposure to organisms causes the body to produce antibodies which aid in supplying greater resistance.
- Pathogens cause infections when they invade, and because of low resistance, overpower the body's immune system.

UNIVERSAL PRECAUTIONS

- **Universal precautions** are a set of practices for use with all patients to prevent the spread of disease.
- Because of the arrival of the human immunodeficiency virus (HIV) and an increase in hepatitis B, C, and D viruses, the Centers for Disease Control (CDC) requires that universal precautions be used at all times.
- **Universal precautions** comprise safe practices that aid in protection from blood and body substances that may contain infection.
- These precautions are descibed as universal because they are employed with every patient.
- Because of the lethal nature of some pathogens, it is necessary that health care providers practice universal precautions.

STANDARD PRECAUTIONS

FOR INFECTION CONTROL

Wash Hands (Plain soap)
Wash after touching **blood**, **body fluids**, **secretions**, **excretions**, and **contaminated items**.
Wash immediately **after gloves are removed** and **between patient contacts**.
Avoid transfer of microorganisms to other patients or environments.

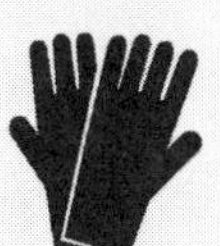

Wear Gloves
Wear when touching **blood**, **body fluids**, **secretions**, **excretions**, and **contaminated items**.
Put on **clean** gloves just **before touching mucous membranes** and **nonintact skin**.
Change gloves between tasks and procedures on the same patient after contact with material that may contain high concentrations of microorganisms. Remove gloves promptly after use, before touching noncontaminated items and environmental surfaces, and before going to another patient, and wash hands immediately to avoid transfer of microorganisms to other patients or environments.

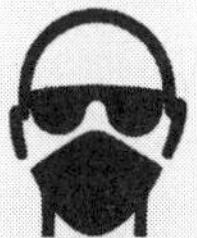

Wear Mask and Eye Protection or Face Shield
Protect mucous membranes of the eyes, nose and mouth during procedures and patient–care activities that are likely to generate **splashes** or **sprays** of **blood**, **body fluids**, **secretions**, or **excretions**.

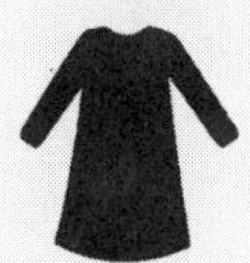

Wear Gown
Protect skin and prevent soiling of clothing during procedures that are likely to generate **splashes** or **sprays** of **blood**, **body fluids**, **secretions**, or **excretions**. Remove a soiled gown as promptly as possible and wash hands to avoid transfer of microorganisms to other patients or environments.

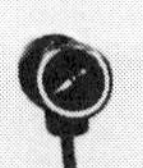

Patient-Care Equipment
Handle used patient–care equipment soiled with **blood**, **body fluids**, **secretions**, or **excretions** in a manner that prevents skin and mucous membrane exposures, contamination of clothing, and transfer of microorganisms to other patients and environments. Ensure that reusable equipment is not used for the care of another patient until it has been appropriately cleaned and reprocessed and single use items are properly discarded.

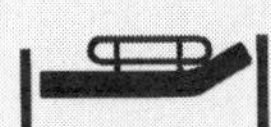

Environmental Control
Follow hospital procedures for routine care, cleaning, and disinfection of environmental surfaces, beds, bedrails, bedside equipment and other frequently touched surfaces.

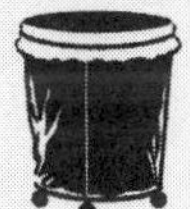

Linen
Handle, transport, and process used linen soiled with **blood**, **body fluids**, **secretions**, or **excretions** in a manner that prevents exposures and contamination of clothing, and avoids transfer of microorganisms to other patients and environments.

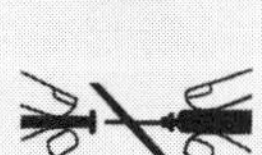

Occupational Health and Bloodborne Pathogens
Prevent injuries when using needles, scalpels, and other sharp instruments or devices; when handling sharp instruments after procedures; when cleaning used instruments; and when disposing of used needles.

Never recap used needles using both hands or any other technique that involves directing the point of a needle toward any part of the body; rather, use either a one-handed "scoop" technique or a mechanical device designed for holding the needle sheath.

Do not remove used needles from disposable syringes by hand, and do not bend, break, or otherwise manipulate used needles by hand. Place used disposable syringes and needles, scalpel blades, and other sharp items in puncture–resistant sharps containers located as close as practical to the area in which the items were used, and place reusable syringes and needles in a puncture–resistant container for transport to the reprocessing area.

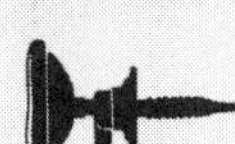

Use **resuscitation devices** as an alternative to mouth–to–mouth resuscitation.

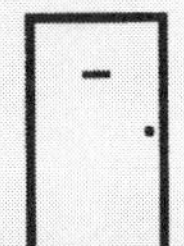

Patient Placement
Use a **private room** for a patient who contaminates the environment or who does not (or cannot be expected to) assist in maintaining appropriate hygiene or environmental control. Consult Infection Control if a private room is not available.

The information on this sign is abbreviated from the HICPAC Recommendations for Isolation Precautions in Hospitals.

Form No. **SPR** BREVIS CORP., 3310 S 2700 E, SLC, UT 84109

CONTACT PRECAUTIONS

(in addition to Standard Precautions)

VISITORS: Report to nurse before entering.

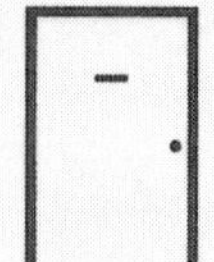

Patient Placement

Private room, if possible. Cohort if private room is not available.

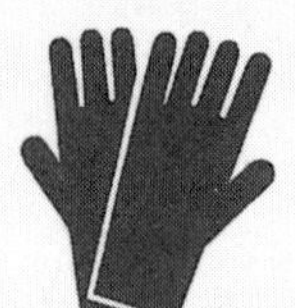

Gloves

Wear gloves when entering the room.
Change gloves after having contact with infective material that may contain high concentrations of microorganisms **(fecal** material and **wound drainage**).
Remove gloves before leaving patient room.

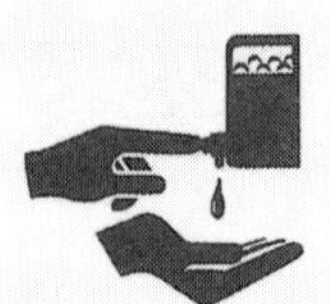

Wash

Wash hands with an **antimicrobial** agent immediately after glove removal .
After glove removal and handwashing, ensure that hands do not touch potentially contaminated environmental surfaces or items in the patient's room to avoid transfer of microorganisms to other patients or environments.

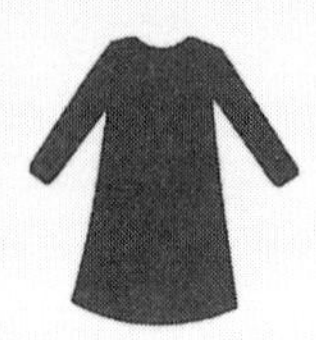

Gown

Wear gown when **entering** the room if you anticipate that your clothing will have substantial contact with the patient, environmental surfaces, or items in the patient's room, or if the patient is **incontinent**, or has **diarrhea**, an **ileostomy**, a **colostomy**, or **wound drainage** not contained by a dressing. **Remove** the gown before leaving the patient's environment and ensure that clothing does not contact potentially contaminated environmental surfaces to avoid transfer of microorganisms to other patients or environments.

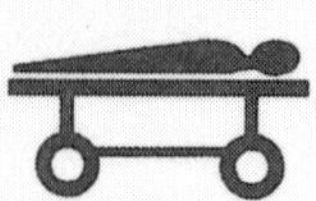

Patient Transport

Limit transport of patient to essential purposes only. During transport, ensure that precautions are maintained to minimize the risk of transmission of microorganisms to other patients and contamination of environmental surfaces and equipment.

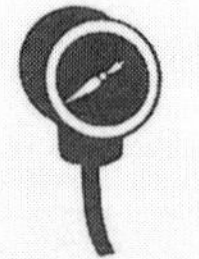

Patient–Care Equipment

Dedicate the use of noncritical patient–care equipment (e.g., stethoscope, sphygmomanometer, bedside commode, electronic rectal thermometer) to a single patient. If common equipment is used, clean and disinfect between patients.

Form No. **CPR** BREVIS CORP., 3310 S 2700 E, SLC, UT 84109

- **Body substances** that may harbor infections include
  - Blood and semen
  - Vaginal fluid
  - Peritoneal fluid
  - Pericardial fluid
  - Pleural fluid
  - Amniotic and sinovial fluid
  - Cerebrospinal fluid
  - Vomit
  - Feces and urine
  - Saliva and sputum
  - Any wound drainage.
- **Body substance isolation** is a term that characterizes all body substances as infectious.
- Specific **methods of isolation** have been denoted for body substances:
  - Hand washing should be executed before and after patient contact and before and after gloving.
  - Gloves should be worn any time contact with body substances is possible.
  - When splashing of fluid is possible, goggles, protective glasses, a face shield, and a mask should be employed.
  - Impenetrable gowns should be worn if substance soiling is possible.
  - Accidental needle sticks should be avoided by using proper disposal receptacles. Do not bend or break needles before disposal.
  - Gloves damaged during the administration of care should be replaced immediately.
  - Always use mouthpieces and resuscitation devices when performing mouth-to-mouth resuscitation.
  - Place all soiled objects in infectious waste trash bags or containers.
- The use of **personal protective equipment** is necessary to protect health care professionals as well as other patients from the transmission of organisms.
- Personal protective equipment includes, but is not limited to, gloves, a gown, a face shield, goggles, and a mask.

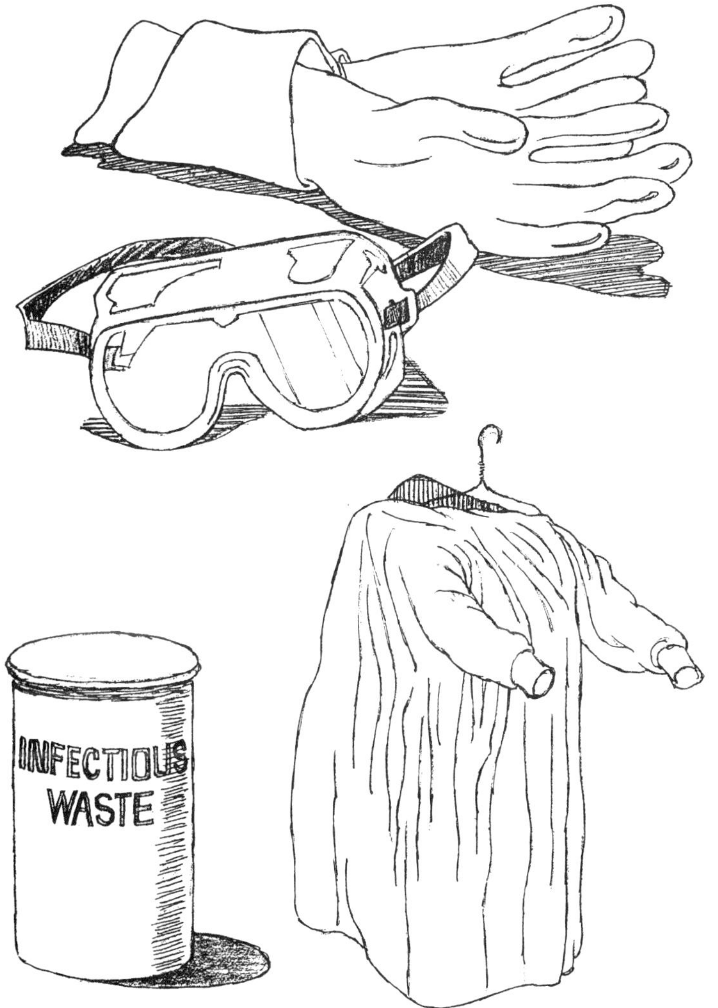

DROPLET PRECAUTIONS

(in addition to Standard Precautions)

VISITORS: Report to nurse before entering.

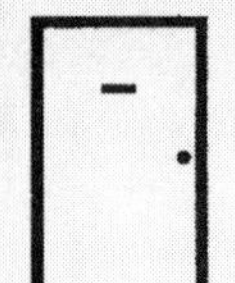

Patient Placement

Private room, if possible. Cohort or maintain spatial separation of **3 feet** from other patients or visitors if private room is not available.

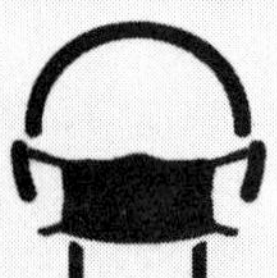

Mask

Wear mask when working within **3 feet** of patient (or upon entering room).

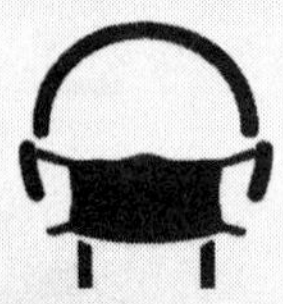

Patient Transport

Limit transport of patient from room to essential purposes only.
Use **surgical mask** on patient during transport.

Form No. **DPR** BREVIS CORP., 3310 S 2700 E, SLC, UT 84109

INFECTION CONTROL PROCEDURES

- Implementation of proper universal precautions and medical asepsis helps control the spread of microorganisms.
- **Medical asepsis** is the process by which pathogens are destroyed after they leave the body.
- The **procedure** used to help destroy organisms through medical asepsis involves soap and water, friction, and disinfection.

Hand-Washing and Gloving Procedures

- Proper hand-washing technique is the **single greatest measure** that can be employed to prevent the spread of disease.
- Hands should be washed before and after putting on gloves and **between contacts** with patients.
- All cuts or **abrasions** on the hands should be covered at all times to prevent infection.

- Fingernails should be short, and wearing jewelry on the hands should be minimal because it harbors microbes.
- Proper hand-washing technique is a medically aseptic procedure.
- There are **various methods** of hand washing differentiated by the length of time involved and the amount of the arm that is scrubbed.
- The full **2-minute technique** usually involves the elbow to the fingertips.
- When scrubbing between patients during general care settings, it is necessary to scrub from the wrist area to the fingertips for at least **30 seconds**.

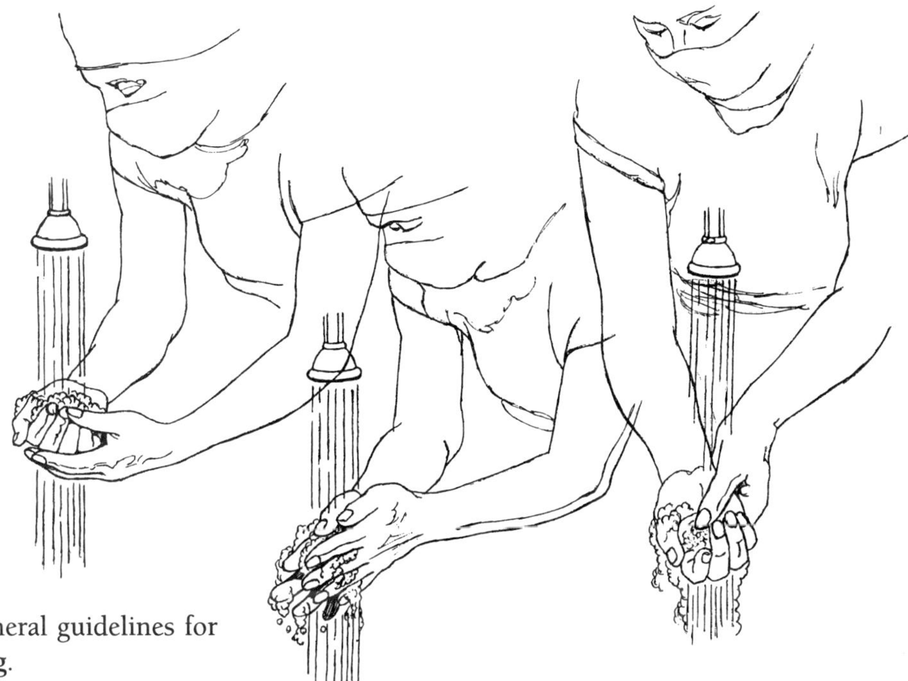

- The following are general guidelines for **aseptic hand washing**.
  1. Turn on the faucet with a paper towel, if necessary. Use a foot control if possible.
  2. Do not lean against or allow clothing to touch the sink.
  3. Using warm water, flowing at a normal rate, and soap, scrub all parts of the hands and fingers.
  4. Always keep the hands lower than the elbows, allowing water to drain down the arms.
  5. Rinse the arms and hands thoroughly.
  6. Turn off the faucet without touching the handles (see step 1).
  7. Dry the hands and arms completely.
  8. Apply a moisturizer if necessary to prevent chafing and abrasions.

- **Gloves** should be worn whenever contact with body substances is possible.
- Gloves should be replaced immediately if a tear develops.
- **Soiled gloves** should be removed using the following method.
  1. With a gloved hand remove the glove of the opposite hand by pulling it down from the cuff and turning it inside out.
  2. Holding the glove you have just removed in the palm of the gloved hand, pull the remaining glove off by reaching inside with the first two fingers and drawing the glove off while turning it inside out.
  3. Both gloves should now be folded together ready to be discarded.

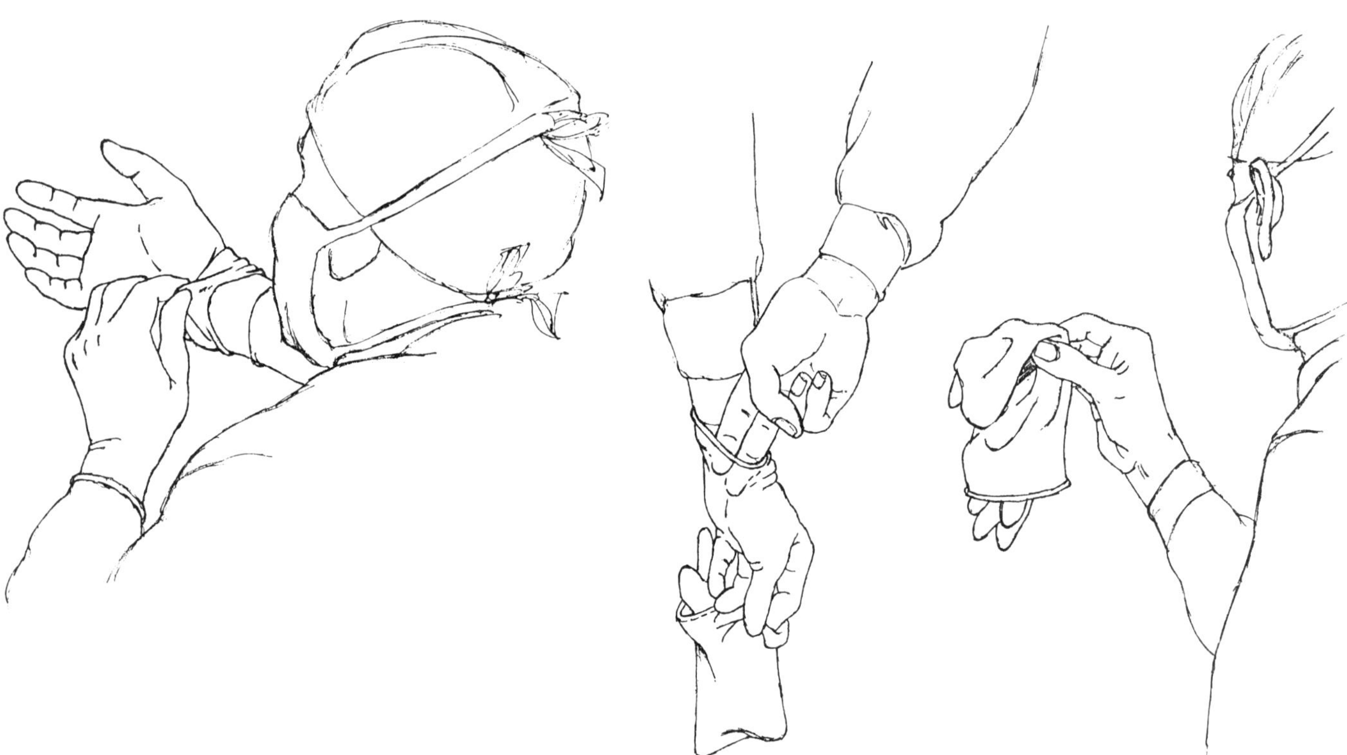

Disinfection and Discarding Refuse

- **Disinfection** is the removal of microorganisms by a mechanical or chemical process.
- Disinfection does not remove the spores of microorganisms.
- **Asepsis** is a common term for disinfection of body surfaces.

- Containers housing disinfectant solution for cleaning purposes should be changed daily.
- All linen, including pillowcases, should be changed between each patient.
- The radiographer should carry soiled or used linen away from his body.
- Used linen **should not be shaken** or moved in a way that may stir up dust carrying pathogens.
- Any item that touches the floor should be discarded because the floor is a resting place for numerous microorganisms.
- **Body fluids** should be disposed of immediately unless they are being kept for analysis.
- **Disposable supplies** should be used whenever possible.
- Supplies that can be reused must be **sterilized** before being used for another patient.
- All equipment should be cleaned with a **disinfectant-dampened** cloth between patients.
- Anything exposed to or contaminated by an infectious organism should be transported in a **sealed container.**
- Cleaning should always start in the least soiled area and conclude in the most soiled area.
- Equipment should not be used if its level of cleanliness is unknown.

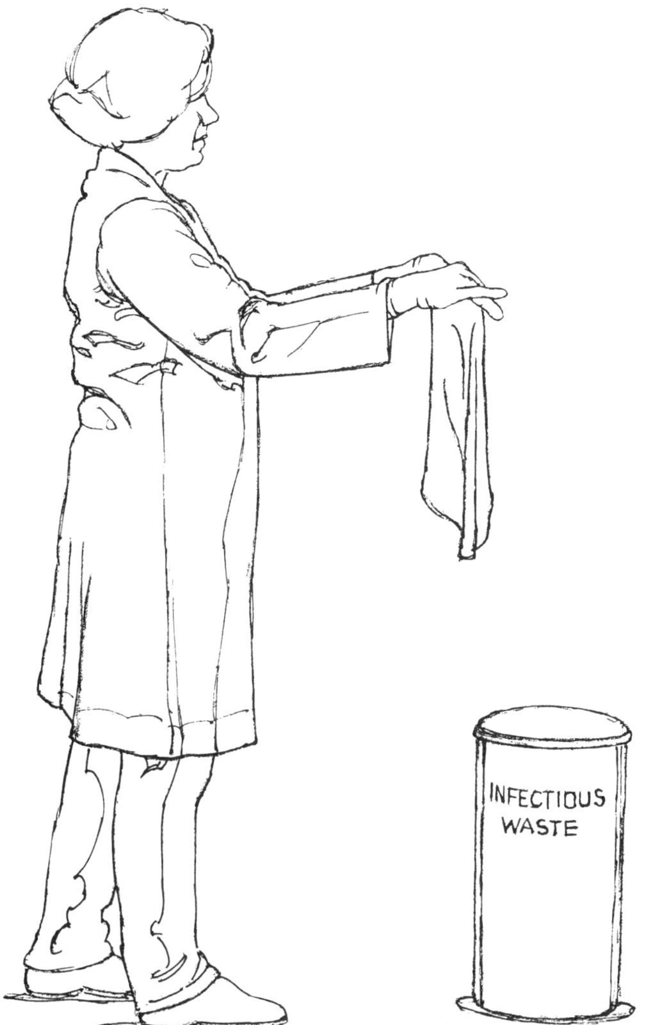

Sharps Disposal

- All sharp instruments, including needles, should be **dropped** in the designated container immediately after use.
- **Sharps containers** should be in the immediate vicinity and labeled as a biohazard.
- Fingers should never enter the container.
- Used needles should not be bent, broken, recapped, or removed from syringes before discarding.
- All containers should be sealed and replaced when they are no more than two-thirds full.

Isolation

- Techniques of isolation are broken into two separate types: category-specific isolation and disease-specific isolation.
- **Category-specific isolation** groups diseases according to their route of transmission.
- **Disease-specific isolation** groups diseases according to the infection control techniques required for specific diseases.

Category-Specific Isolation

- The seven techniques used in category-specific isolation are
  - Acid-fast bacilli (AFB) isolation
  - Blood and body fluid precautions
  - Contact isolation
  - Drainage secretions precautions
  - Enteric precautions
  - Respiratory isolation
  - Strict isolation.

AIRBORNE PRECAUTIONS
(in addition to Standard Precautions)

VISITORS: Report to nurse before entering.

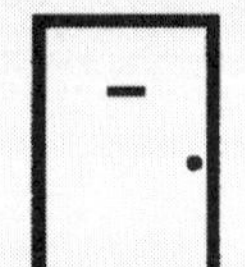

Patient Placement
Use **private room** that has:
Monitored negative air pressure,
6 to 12 air changes per hour,
Discharge of air outdoors or HEPA filtration if recirculated.
Keep room door closed and patient in room.

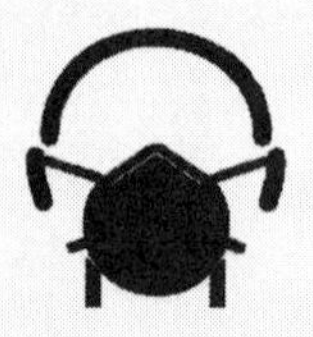

Respiratory Protection
Wear an **N95 respirator** when entering the room of a patient with known or suspected infectious pulmonary **tuberculosis.**
Susceptible persons should not enter the room of patients known or suspected to have **measles** (rubeola) or **varicella** (chickenpox) if other immune caregivers are available. If susceptible persons must enter, they should wear an **N95 respirator.** (Respirator or surgical mask not required if immune to measles and varicella.)

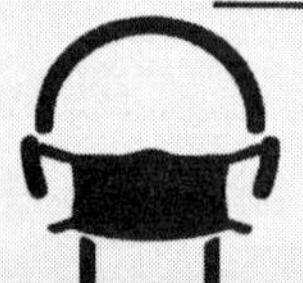

Patient Transport
Limit transport of patient from room to essential purposes only.
Use **surgical mask** on patient during transport.

Form No. **APR** BREVIS CORP., 3310 S 2700 E, SLC, UT 84109 © 1996 Brevis Corp.

- **AFB isolation** is used to prevent contamination via small particles in the air. It is employed chiefly when treating active tuberculosis.
- It is necessary to use a specialized respiratory mask, a gown, and gloves. Room ventilation is also a concern.
- **Blood and body fluid** precautions, as stated before, are used to prevent the spread of microorganisms through contact with contaminated body fluids.
- Protective equipment used for blood and body fluid isolation includes gloves, a gown, a mask, and eyewear if splashing is possible.
- **Contact isolation** prevents the transmission of highly infectious diseases via direct or close contact with the host.
- Mask, gloves, a gown, and possibly eyewear may be needed when treating a patient using contact isolation precautions.
- **Drainage and secretion precautions** involve prevention of infection through contact with body secretions or drainage.
- It is necessary to wear gloves and a gown.
- **Enteric precautions** are specific for direct or indirect contact involving exposure to fecal material.
- Protective barriers should include gloves, a gown, and protective eyewear if splashing is a possiblity.
- **Respiratory isolation** is used to prevent droplet transmission.
- Protective barriers for respiratory isolation include a mask and gloves.
- **Strict isolation** is applied in order to prevent transmission of very contagious infections which may be spread via the air or direct contact.
- Strict isolation may also be employed to prevent the spread of microorganisms to patients who may be susceptible to infection. This form of isolation also has been termed **reverse** or **protective isolation**.
- Protective equipment required usually consists of gloves, a mask, a gown, and protective eyewear.

Disease-Specific Isolation

- **Disease-specific isolation** is contingent on finding the cause of a particular disease.
- Forms of protection depend on the disease and how it can be transmitted.
- Consideration is also given to the ability of the patient to participate in the isolation procedure.

Considerations for the Imaging Professional

- Strict attention should be given to all signs and notices regarding the specific method of isolation the patient may be in.
- Lead aprons should be covered with a non-permeable gown when personal protection is necessary and splash contamination is possible.
- Protective **plastic coverings** should be used with all radiographic cassettes that may come into contact with infectious substances.
- Two technologists should work together employing the **clean/contaminated technologist method**.

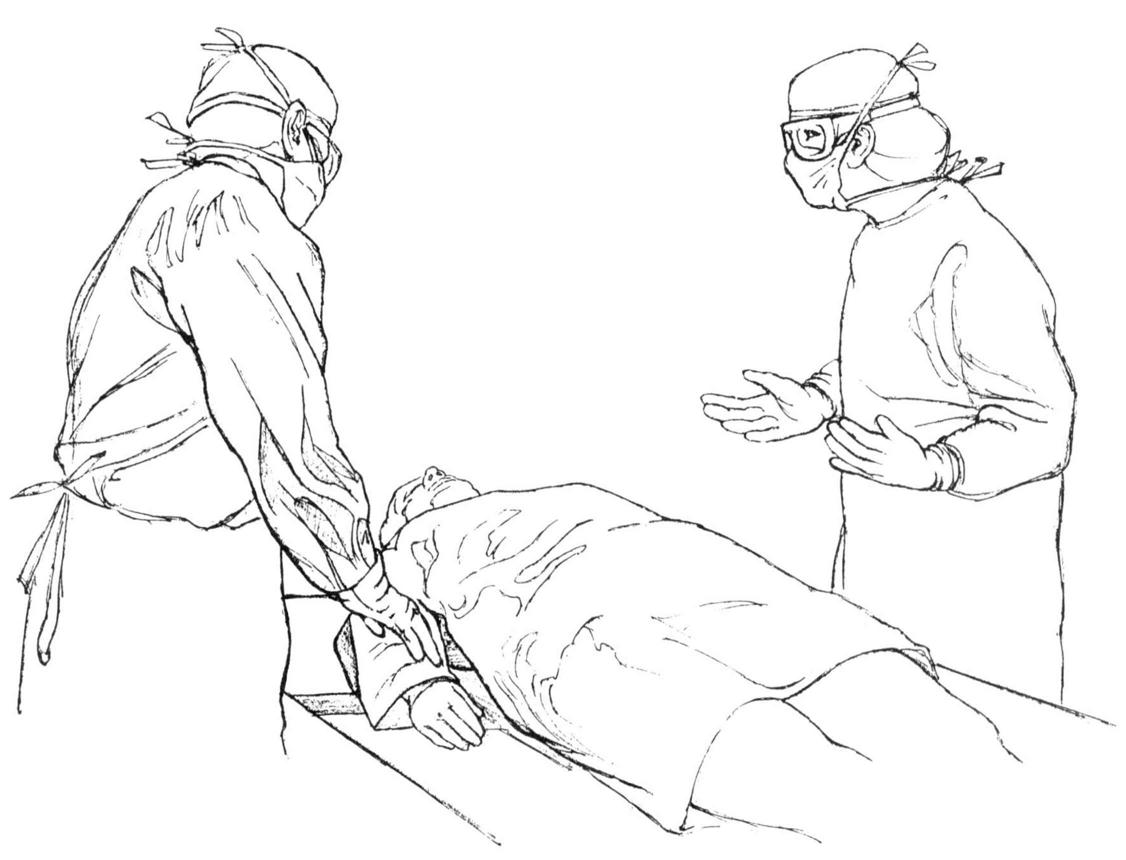

The clean/contaminated method requires that the clean technologist handle the equipment and cassette (when outside the protective plastic covering).
The contaminated technologist handles all equipment that comes into contact with the patient and positions the patient when necessary.

- All portable radiographic equipment should be **disinfected** immediately before and after entering and exiting the patient's room.
- It is imperative that contaminated equipment not be moved from one area to another.
- When transporting patients who are in isolation precautions it is essential that the technologist employ all the necessary **protective barriers.**
- Wheelchairs or gurneys used to transport patients should be disinfected outside the patient's room.
- All used linen should be immediately discarded in the nearest receptacle.
- The imaging room should be completely disinfected immediately after the procedure is completed.

Chapter 4 Review Questions

1. **The greatest accumulation of microorganisms occurs on which of the following?**
   a. the patient's bed
   b. any open wound
   c. the floor of a room
   d. the bed linen
2. **Which of the following is used to denote a disease-causing organism?**
   a. infection
   b. pathogen
   c. microorganism
   d. all of the above
3. **Which of the four main types of pathogens has DNA, has RNA, and is single-celled?**
   a. bacteria
   b. viruses
   c. fungi
   d. molds

4. **The coating around the nucleus of a bacteria that acts as a protective barrier is called a**
   a. fomite.
   b. spore.
   c. vector.
   d. protozoan.

5. **During which stage of infection does the microorganism start to reproduce and infection begin?**
   a. latent period
   b. incubation period
   c. disease period
   d. convalescent period

6. **During which stage of infection is the host most communicable?**
   a. latent period
   b. incubation period
   c. disease period
   d. convalescent period

7. **Which of the following is a means of spreading infection?**
   a. contact
   b. vehicle
   c. air
   d. all of the above

8. **The spread of infection via contaminated food is which kind of infection?**
   a. contact
   b. vehicle
   c. air
   d. vector

9. **In defending against specific outside organisms the immune system responds by forming**
   a. antibodies.
   b. pathogens.
   c. histamines.
   d. antigens.

10. **Which of the following is not a type of immunity?**
    a. pathogenic
    b. natural
    c. acquired
    d. active

11. **A set of practices that aid in disease prevention are termed**
    a. universal precautions.
    b. surgical asepsis.
    c. medical asepsis.
    d. sterile technique.

12. **Which of the following should be done when disposing of a needle?**
    a. recap
    b. break
    c. remove from the syringe
    d. all of the above
    e. none of the above

13. **The process by which pathogens are destroyed after they leave the body is known as**
    a. universal precautions.
    b. surgical asepsis.
    c. medical asepsis.
    d. sterile technique.

14. **The single greatest measure that can be utilized to prevent the spread of infection is**
    a. proper discarding of refuse.
    b. proper handwashing technique.
    c. proper disinfection of radiographic cassettes.
    d. employing gloves when disinfecting equipment.

15. **Which of the following can remove microorganisms but not their spores?**
    I. sterilization
    II. disinfection
    III. mechanical disinfection

    a. only I and II
    b. only II and III
    c. only I and III
    d. I, II, and III

16. **Which form of isolation precautions is specific to exposure to fecal material?**
    a. drainage/secretion precautions
    b. contact isolation precautions
    c. enteric isolation precautions
    d. strict isolation precautions

17. **Which of the following are used to protect immunosuppressed patients from pathogens?**
    a. drainage/secretion precautions
    b. contact isolation precautions
    c. enteric isolation precautions
    d. strict isolation precautions

18. **Dropping a needle into a sharps container aids in which of the following?**
    a. ease in emptying the container
    b. ease in removing the needle from the syringe
    c. decreased possibility of a needle stick
    d. all of the above

19. **A bandage removed from an open wound should be considered**
    a. infected.
    b. contaminated.
    c. sterile.
    d. aseptic.

20. **Which of the following is required when x-raying a patient under respiratory isolation precautions?**
    I. **The imaging professional should wear a mask.**
    II. **The patient should wear a mask.**
    III. **Hands should be washed before and after x-raying the patient.**

    a. only I
    b. only II
    c. only III
    d. I, II, and III

CHAPTER 5

Surgical Asepsis

- **Surgical asepsis** describes a process used to keep an area or object free of organisms by destroying the pathogens and their spores.
- The procedure used to accomplish surgical asepsis is termed **sterilization**.
- An object is considered **sterile** if it is free of microorganisms and unable to produce any life forms.
- There are four different **methods** of sterilization, including autoclaving (steam under pressure), dry heat, gas, and chemical measures.
- The **autoclave** or steam-under-pressure technique is the safest, most efficient method of sterilization.
- **Chemical** sterilization is becoming more popular as heat-sensitive high-technology instruments become more commonplace in surgical procedures.
- The **four fundamental rules** of surgical asepsis are as follows:
  - Know what is sterile
  - Know what is unsterile
  - Separate the sterile from the unsterile
  - Rectify contamination as soon as possible.
- Sterile packages should always be dated and labeled to inform the user as to when the contents were sterilized.
- When a sterile surface comes into contact with something that is unsterile, the sterile surface becomes contaminated.
- Moving air currents, shaking linen, and unnecessary speech can stir up microorganisms which may land on a sterile field unnecessarily.

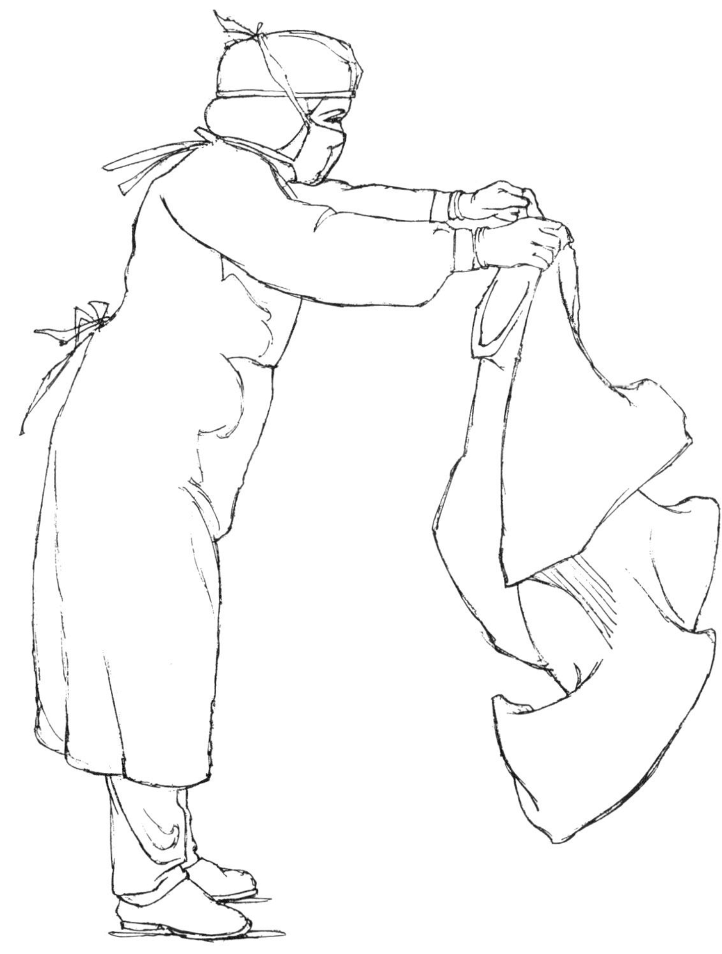

- The **sterile field** is a specific area that is protected from microorganisms and on which only sterile objects should be placed.
- If an item cannot be sterilized because of size or complexity, it should be disinfected using strict medical asepsis.
- Noncommercial products sterilized within the hospital should be stored separately from nonsterile packages.
- Some sort of **indicator** or label should be placed on a sterile packages to denote its shelf life.
- If a sterile field or surface becomes **contaminated**, it is imperative the condition be rectified by employing the following measures:
    1. Remove any contaminated object from the region.
    2. Cover the contaminant with a sterile towel if necessary.
    3. Discard the contaminant or, if the entire field has been compromised, reestablish a sterile field.
- It is important that if one does not know whether something is sterile, they should assume that it is unsterile.
- If contamination is suspected, assume that it has occurred and rectify the situation immediately.

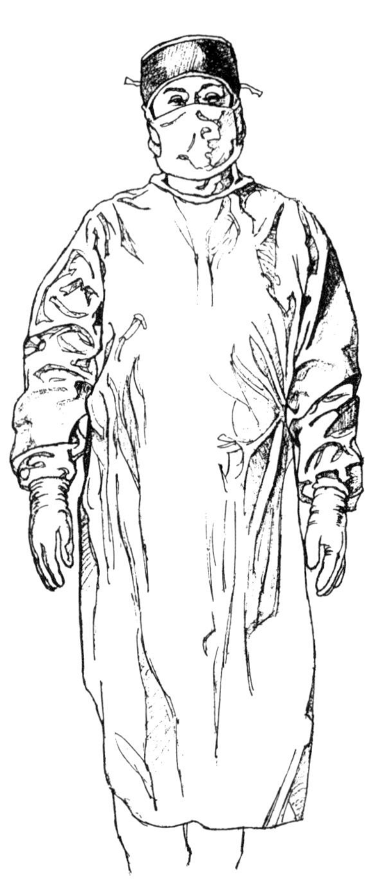

STANDARDS OF SURGICAL TECHNIQUE

- Anything that is in contact with a sterile field must be sterile.
- **Sterile gowns** are considered sterile only in the front from the chest to the level of the sterile field.
- **Sleeves** are considered sterile from 2 inches above the elbow to the wrist.
- Only the **top of a sterile drape** is considered sterile.
- A 1-inch area around all open packages and the table is considered unsterile.
- When placing the contents in a sterile field, they should be carefully placed in the midportion of the field.

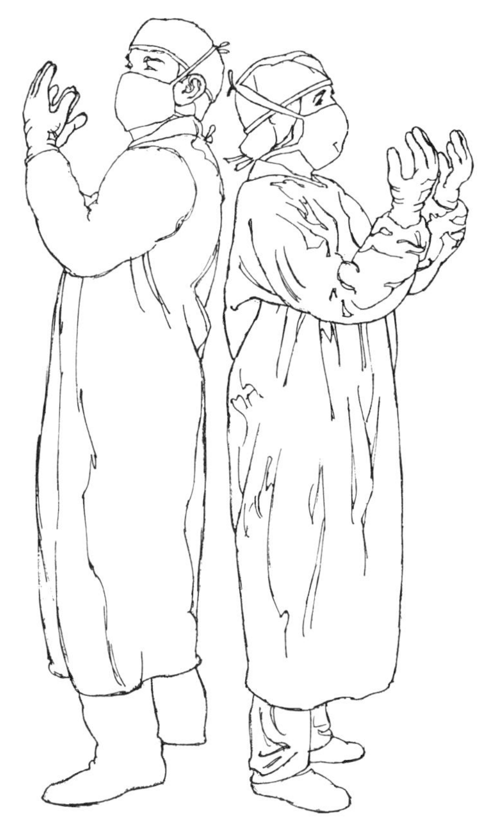

- When **passing sterile surfaces**, one should always keep the sterile field in sight.
- Two sterile people should pass each other back to back in order to maintain the sterile field.
- Hands and arms considered sterile should be kept above **waist level** at all times.
- Anything that hangs below the level of the table or waist is considered unsterile.
- The sterile field should be monitored at all times.
- The floor is considered the **most impure** portion of the room. If anything falls onto the floor it is no longer sterile.

SURGICAL SCRUB

- The **surgical scrub technique** is similar to the aseptic hand-washing procedure.
- The process of turning on the faucet, rinsing, drying, and turning off the faucet is the same as previously noted.
- The **duration** of the surgical scrub is from 5 to 10 minutes.
- It is essential that antimicrobial soap, a scrub brush or sponge, the minimum prescribed strokes, and friction be employed.
- The scrub should cover a **region** from approximately 2 inches above the elbow to the fingertips.
- The **nails** should be cleaned with a minimum of 30 brush strokes and the remaining skin with at least 20 brush strokes.
- Thorough rinsing is important to remove soap and dead skin.
- When **drying** the scrubbed area, the fingertips should be dried completely before the forearm is dried.
- One should move up the arm, being careful not to retrace any portion that has already been dried, as this may cause contamination.

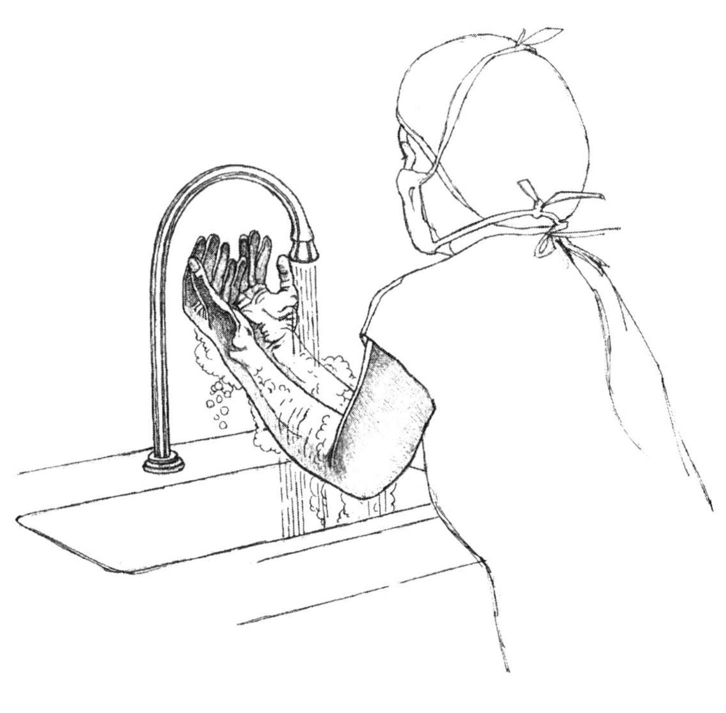

SURGICAL GOWNING

- The following **procedure** should be utilized when donning a sterile gown:

  Pick the gown up off the table and allow it to fall open lengthwise.

  Hold the gown by the inside, close to the shoulder seams.

  Carefully **slide both hands** into the arm holes simultaneously.

  Do not allow the hands to be lowered past shoulder level or advance past the cuff of the gown if sterile gloves will also be worn.

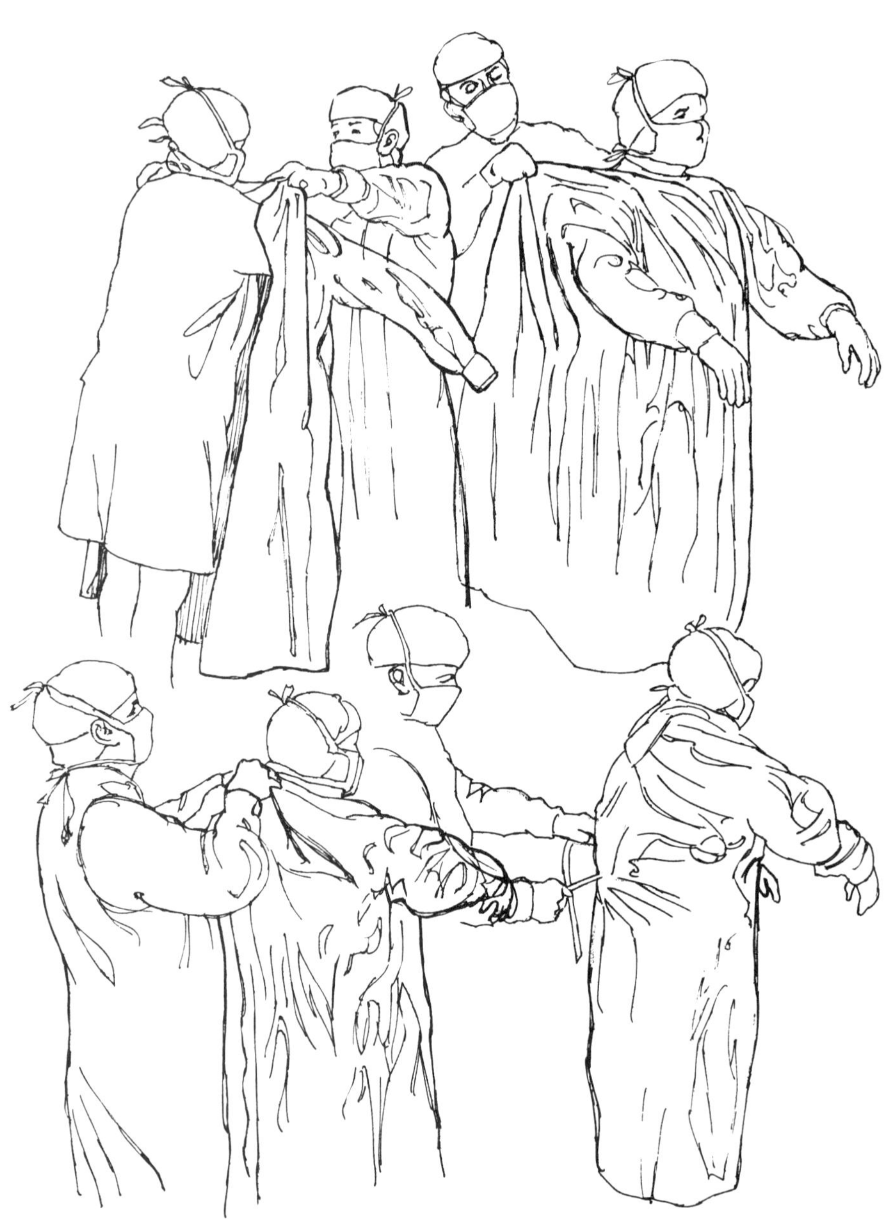

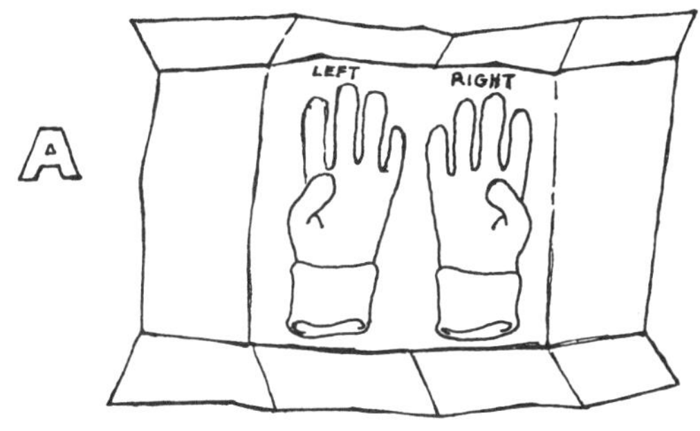

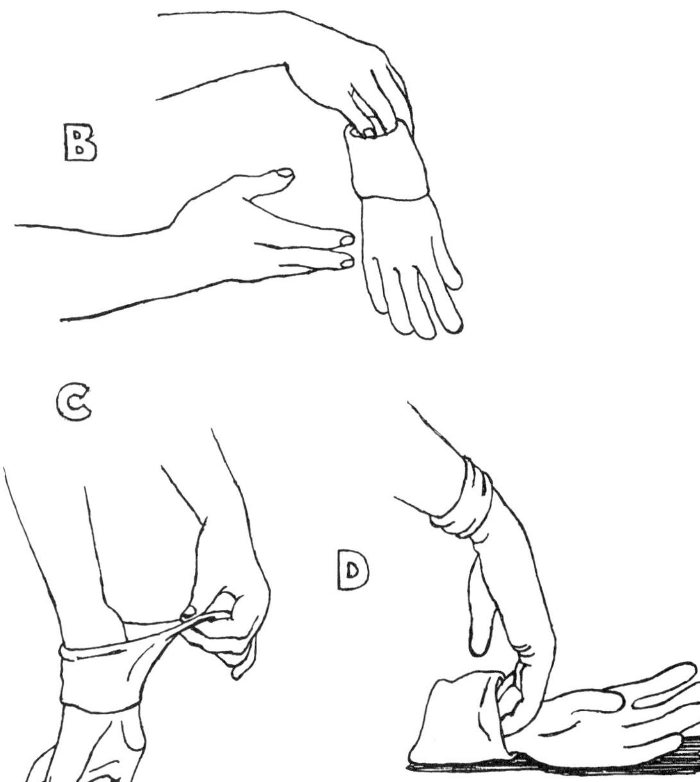

STERILE GLOVES

- The two methods used to apply sterile gloves are the open method and the closed method.
- The **open method** should be employed whenever one is also required to wear a sterile gown, as it allows for the integrity of the cuff of the gown to be maintained.
- The **closed method** is used most frequently in the imaging department and is the technique of choice when only sterile gloves are necessary for the procedure.
- The following is the closed **method** of applying sterile gloves:
  - Pick up the glove of your dominant hand by the outside of the cuff.
  - Glove your dominant hand first, touching only the outside of the cuff.
  - It is not important for the glove to be perfectly placed on the hand, as it will be adjusted later.
  - Pick up the glove of the remaining hand under the fold of the cuff.
  - Pull the glove over the remaining hand.
  - It is important when adjusting the gloves that only the outside portion be touched.
  - If the gloves tear, remove them and start the procedure over again.

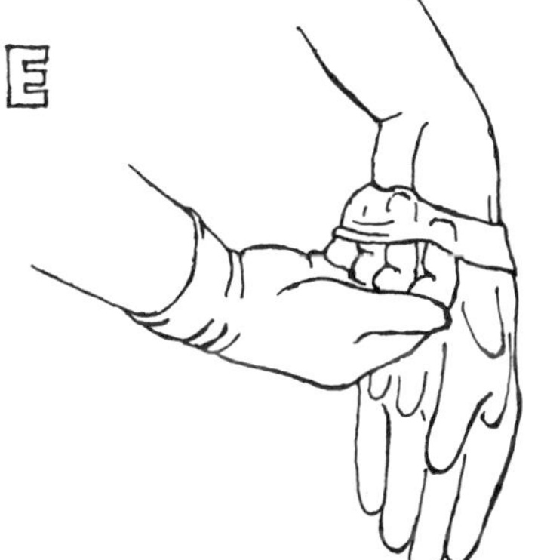

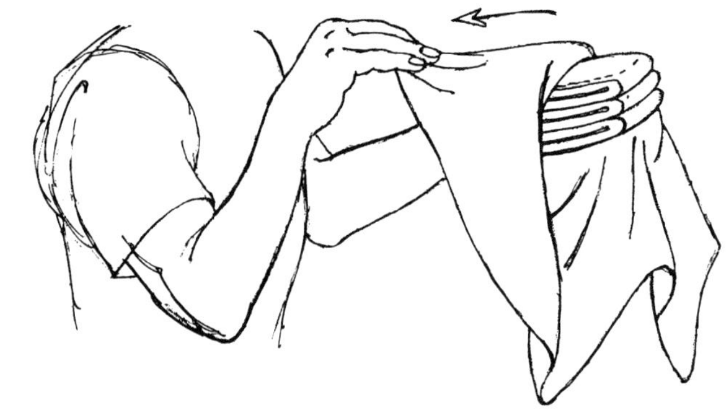

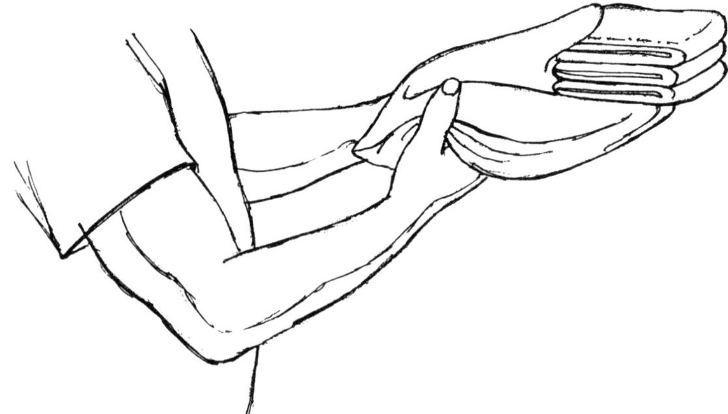

OPENING STERILE PACKAGES

- Expiration dates should be checked before opening a package to ensure that the contents are sterile.
- Radiographers should **wash** their hands before beginning to open a sterile package.
- Sterile packages should be unwrapped away from the body.
- Touch only the outside of the wrapper. This area will not be considered sterile.
- The sterile package should be placed in the middle of the area it will be occupying.
- The package should be opened by lifting the distal flap and pulling down toward the edge of the table.
- The lateral flaps should be removed next, followed by the proximal flap.
- It is important that the last flap removed be the proximal flap, which prevents one from reaching directly over the contents of the package.
- One should always face the sterile field and slowly move around it if necessary when unwrapping the package.
- A distance of 1 foot should be maintained if an unsterile person is moving around a sterile field.

SKIN PREPARATION

- **Skin preparation** prevents microorganisms from entering a surgical incision.
- It may be necessary to **shave** all hair from the area that is to be prepared.
- If shaving is essential in helping to prevent infection, a physician's order must be obtained.
- A **4-inch area** around the site should be shaved. It is important to shave in the same direction as the hair grows.
- Skin preparation should involve a **two-step process**; the first step is mechanical and the second chemical.

- **Mechanical preparation** is achieved with a scrub using a sponge with antimicrobial solution and sterile water brought to room temperature.
- Sterile gloves must be worn for the process.
- As in any skin preparation, friction is important in the process.
- It is important to clean from the **inside** of the field to the **outside** of the field.
- Once the field has been lathered and the edges reached, the process should be **repeated with another sponge.**
- The mechanical portion of the scrub should last for at least 5 minutes and no more than 10 minutes.
- The skin should be rinsed with sterile water and any excess wiped off, always moving from the inside of the field outward.
- The **chemical method** involves the use of antiseptic solution.
- The antiseptic solution should be applied moving from the **inner portion of the area outward.**
- Only **one pass** should be made per sponge or swab when applying antiseptic solution.

STERILE DRAPING

- The **surgical draping procedure** is used to set up and maintain a sterile field.
- Sterile towels or disposable drapes are often used.

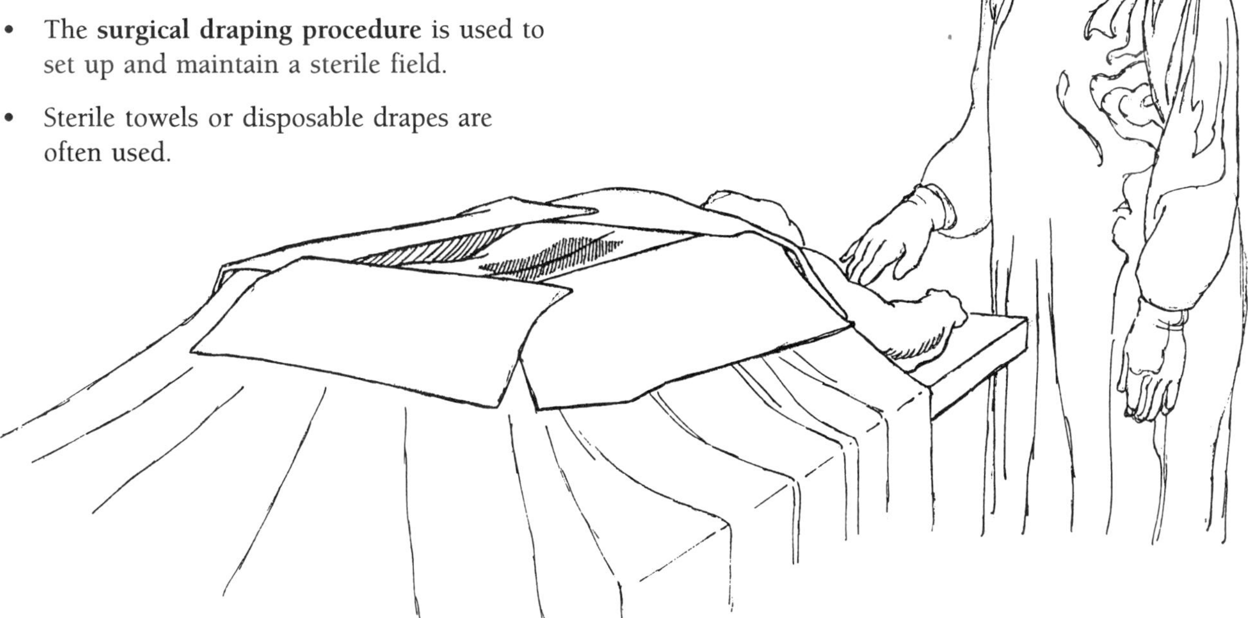

- The person performing the draping procedure should **cautiously open** the package of sterile towels and then don sterile gloves.
- In the imaging department the patient is usually covered with sterile drapes in preparation for a procedure requiring strict surgical asepsis.
- **Survey** the site to be draped before beginning to place the drapes on the patient.
- Do not flip or shake open the drape. Instead, allow gravity to unfold it.
- When draping a nonsterile area, drape from the **outside of the field toward the inside.**
- When draping an area that has been prepared for a procedure, drape the area of interest first and then proceed to the outer edges.
- If the sterility of a drape is unknown, consider it contaminated.
- Drapes should not be moved once they have been placed on a patient.

Chapter 5 Review Questions

1. **Surgical asepsis refers to the removal of which of the following?**
   a. all microorganisms
   b. all microorganisms and their spores which may produce life
   c. pathogens
   d. infection
2. **Which of the following is the same as sterilization?**
   a. medical asepsis
   b. antisepsis
   c. surgical asepsis
   d. all of the above
3. **Which of the following is the autoclave method of sterilization?**
   a. steam under pressure
   b. dry heat
   c. ultraviolet light
   d. ethylene gas

4. **Any item that will penetrate the skin or a mucous membrane must undergo which of the following?**
   a. disinfection
   b. a friction wash with soap and water
   c. sterilization
   d. cleanliness

5. **Which of the following can contaminate a sterile area?**
   a. air currents
   b. unnecessary talking
   c. shaking linen
   d. all of the above
   e. only a and c

6. **If the sterility of an object is unknown, which of the following should be done?**
   a. Ask the physician if it is alright to use the object.
   b. Use the object as long as it has not been dropped on the floor.
   c. Consider the object unsterile and do not use it.
   d. Clean the object with a disinfectant or antimicrobial before using it.

7. **Which of the following is considered to be the unsterile portion of a table which contains sterile instruments?**
   a. the sides and approximately one inch around the table-top
   b. the sides only
   c. one inch around the table top only
   d. All of the table would be considered sterile.

8. **Which of the following regions of a sterile gown are considered sterile?**
   a. from the shoulders to the hips to include the arms
   b. the entire front and back of the gown
   c. from the neck to the waist including the arms
   d. in front from the chest to the level of the table and the arms from 2 inches above the elbow to the wrist

9. **Two people in sterile attire should pass each other in which of the following ways?**
   a. front to back
   b. back to front
   c. back to back
   d. front to front

10. **Which of the following would be considered unsterile?**
    a. the draped sides of a table
    b. hands in sterile gloves hanging at the waist
    c. the back of a sterile gown
    d. all of the above

11. **Which of the following is the normal duration of a surgical scrub?**
    a. 1–2 minutes
    b. 3–5 minutes
    c. 5–10 minutes
    d. 10–15 minutes

12. **Which of the methods should be employed when placing sterile gloves on over a sterile gown?**
    a. open method
    b. closed method
    c. sterile method
    d. aseptic method

13. **Which of the following should be examined first when using a sterile package?**
    a. the way the package is folded
    b. the type of material used to wrap the package
    c. the expiration date
    d. the way the package is taped

14. **What is the correct sequence when unwrapping a sterile package?**
    a. Remove the lateral flaps first, followed by the proximal flap and then the distal flap.
    b. Remove the distal flap first, followed by the lateral flaps and then the proximal flap.
    c. Remove the proximal flap first, followed by the lateral flap and then the distal flap.
    d. Remove the lateral flaps first, followed by the distal flap and then proximal flap.

15. **What is the minimum accepted distance one should keep from a sterile table?**
    a. 6 in.
    b. 1 ft
    c. 2 ft
    d. 3 ft

16. **When preparing skin for a sterile procedure, one should**
    a. wear sterile gloves.
    b. scrub the area with antimicrobial soap.
    c. apply an antiseptic.
    d. do all of the above.

17. **When draping a patient for a sterile procedure, one should drape**
    a. from the right to the left of the area of interest.
    b. the area of interest first and then proceed to the outer edges of the area.
    c. from the left to the right of the area of interest.
    d. the outer edges of the area and then the area of interest.

18. **If you suspect the radiologist has contaminated her glove, which of the following would be the proper course of action?**
    a. Ignore the contamination. You should not make the physician aware that that her glove is contaminated.
    b. Tell her after you have finished with the procedure.
    c. Keep it to yourself, after all, you only suspect her glove is contaminated.
    d. Make the radiologist aware of the possible contamination immediately and provide her with a new package of sterile gloves.

Acute Care Situations

CHAPTER 6

ACUTE CARE SITUATIONS

- Acute care situations can easily occurr in the imaging department because many of the patients are very ill and may have arrived from the emergency room or hospital ward.

CARDIAC ARREST

- **Cardiac arrest** is the term used to describe loss of heart function.
- **Cardiopulmonary arrest** describes loss of cardiac and respiratory functions.
- **Causes** of cardiopulmonary or cardiac arrest may be the following:
  Myocardial infarct
  Ventricular fibrillation
  Trauma and/or infection
  Toxicity.
- **Myocardial infarct (MI)** is the most common cause of cardiac arrest.
- MI results from a clot (or clots) in the coronary artery (or arteries) that causes ischemia and then death to the heart muscle.
- **Ventricular fibrillation** is usually caused by ventricular tachycardia.
- **Tachycardia** occurs when the myocardium contracts normally but at an elevated rate.
- **Trauma** situations such as burns, head injuries, central nervous system injuries, and accidents in which a great loss of blood has occurred may also cause cardiac arrest.
- Conditions such as pneumonia or injuries to the lungs that result in a lack of oxygen lead to **hypoventilation** which can cause cardiac arrest.

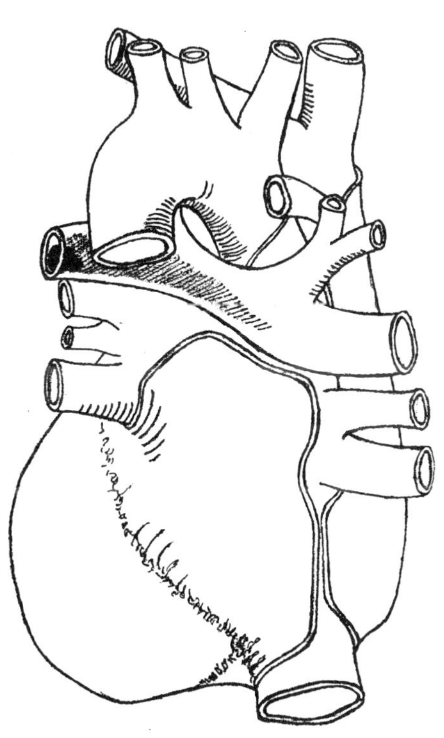

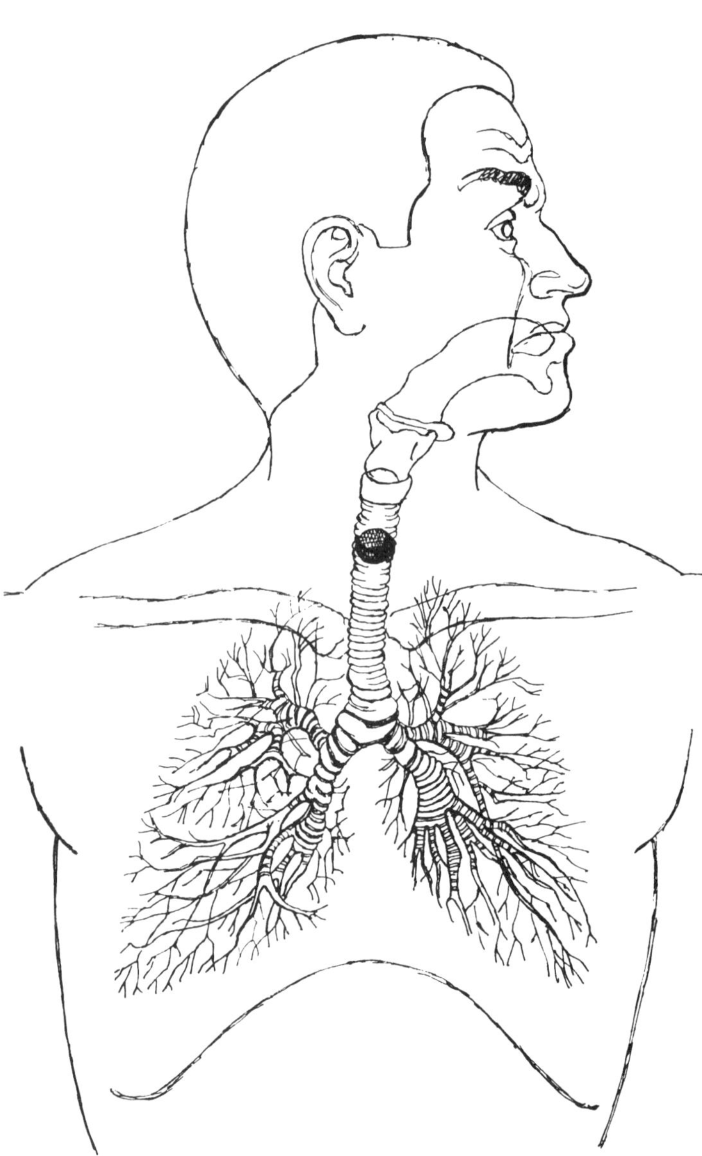

- **Hypoventilation** occurs when the air passage (or passages) are obstructed.

- **Toxicity** may be due to a metabolic imbalance or to drug intoxication.

- **Signs** of cardiopulmonary or cardiac arrest may include
  - Vomiting and/or seizure
  - Lack of a pulse
  - Incontinence or defecation
  - Pale, cool, damp skin
  - Lack of respiration
  - Cyanosis.

- **Cyanosis** is due to a loss of capillary circulation and is manifested as a bluish or grayish-yellow skin tone.

- **Cardiopulmonary resuscitation (CPR)** should be started on any patient in whom cardiac failure is present.

- There are three basic steps when preforming **CPR**:
  - A. Assess the patient's airway for obstruction.
  - B. Start rescue breathing.
  - C. Begin cardiac compressions to circulate the blood.

AIRWAY OBSTRUCTION AND RESPIRATORY FAILURE

- **Airway obstruction** is usually caused by a foreign body obstructing the larynx, trachea, or bronchus.

- **Respiratory distress** is characterized by inability of the lungs to properly oxygenate the blood.

- **Respiratory failure** is an inability of the lungs to oxygenate the blood.

- **Causes** of airway obstruction include
  - A foreign body (dentures, food, etc.)
  - Aspiration (due to vomiting and lack of a gag and/or cough reflex).

- **Symptoms** of respiratory distress are
  - Labored breathing
  - Flared nostrils
  - Tachypnea or bradypnea
  - Headache
  - Cyanosis or diaphoresis
  - Anxiety and/or altered consciousness.

- **Tachypnea** is indicated by a rapid rate of respiration.
- **Bradypnea** is evidenced by abnormally slow respiration.
- **Diaphoresis** is the term used to describe unusual perspiration.
- The **Heimlich maneuver** is used to dislodge foreign bodies from an adult patient's larynx or bronchus.
- **Resuscitation** or ventilation can be accomplished by using the basic CPR techniques.
- The **finger sweep** is usually used to dislodge a foreign object from the throat of an adult.

PULMONARY EMBOLISM

- **Pulmonary embolism** is a blockage in the pulmonary artery (or arteries) due to a thrombus (or thrombi).
- A **thrombus** that leads to an embolism, a thromboembolism, is a clot that loosens and moves.
- **Causes** of pulmonary embolism include
  - Surgery
  - Trauma, especially in the long bones
  - Pathology
  - Poor diet and smoking.
- Oxygen, intravenous fluids, and medications are administered in most situations.
- The following **symptoms** may be observed:
  - Substernal chest pain
  - Shortness of breath and/or cough
  - Dyspnea or tachypnea
  - Cyanosis
  - Hypotension.
- Resulting **complications** due to pulmonary embolism include
  - Pulmonary infarct
  - Atelectasis
  - Pulmonary hypertension
  - Shock
  - Recurrent embolism
  - Death.

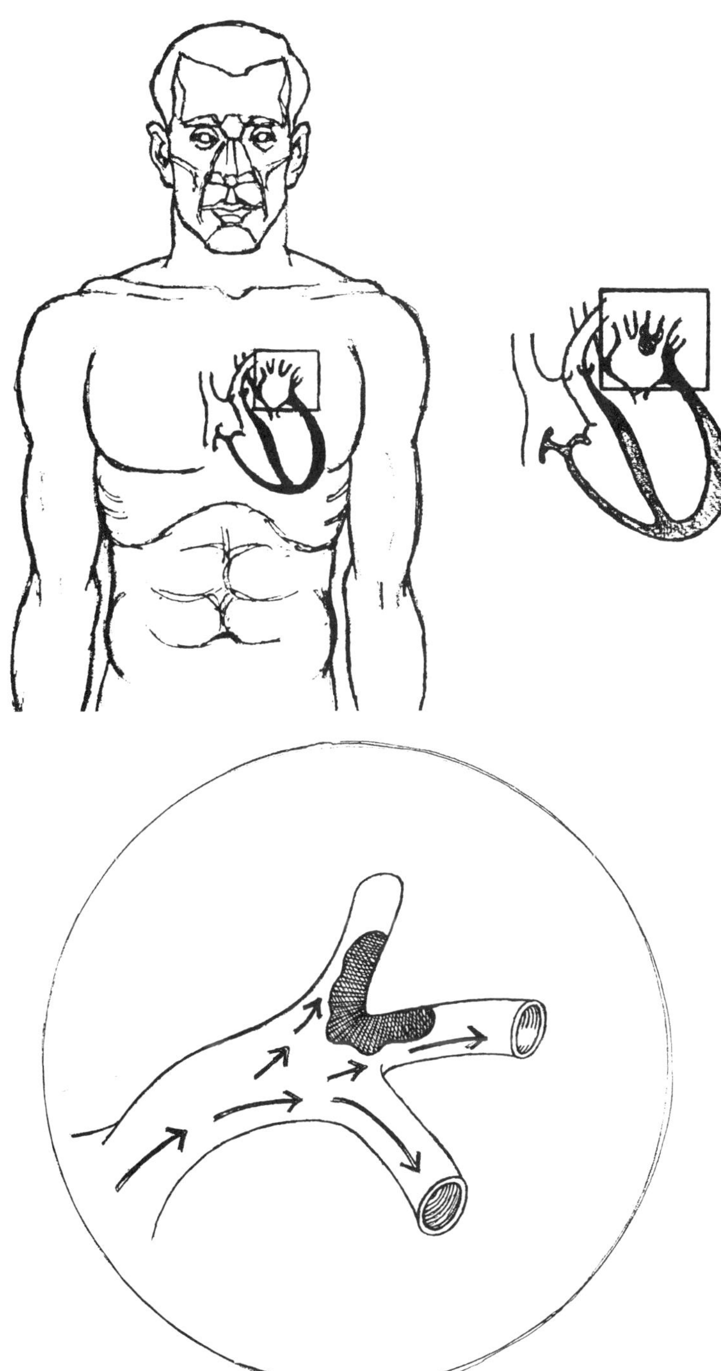

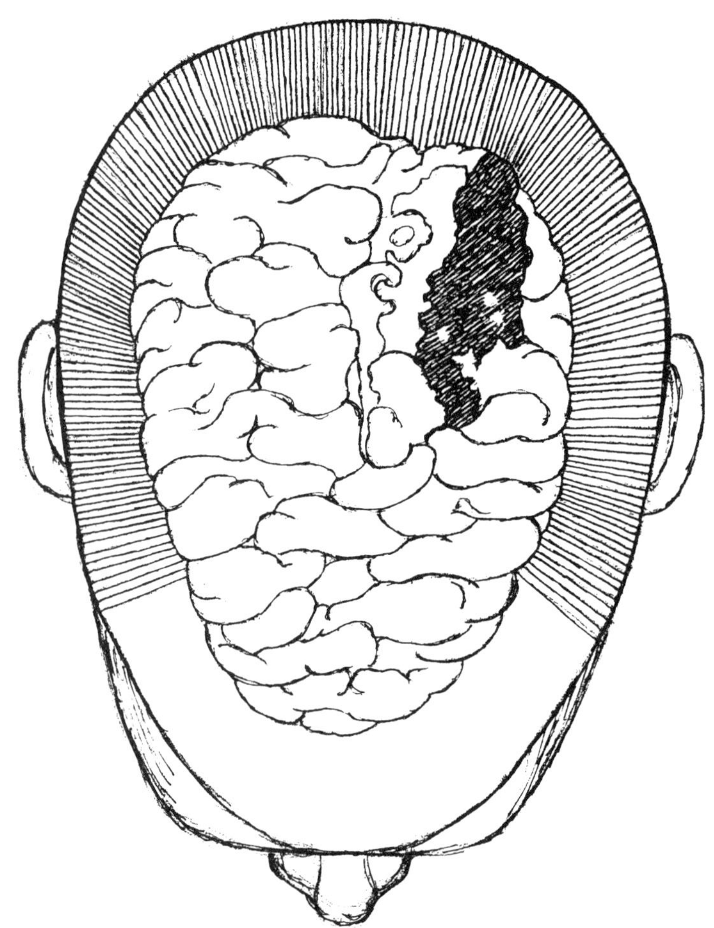

STROKE OR CARDIOVASCULAR ACCIDENT (CVA)

- **Stroke** results from a lack of blood flow to the brain that causes ischemia.
- **Ischemia** is the death of a tissue due to lack of oxygen.
- **Causes** of CVA may be hemorrhage, stenosis, embolism, or thrombosis.
- **Symptoms of CVA** depend on the extent and location of the damage.
- **Signs** may involve any of the following:
  Altered mental state and consciousness
  Bilateral or unilateral numbness
  Bilateral or unilateral paralysis
  Pupil disparity
  Incontinence
  Inability to communicate
  Hypertension
  Dysphagia
  Nausea and/or vomiting.
- A patient with a possible CVA should never be left unattended.
- Vital signs should be assessed frequently.
- **Preparation** should be made for airway ventilation, suction, intravenous fluids, and possible CPR.

SEIZURES

- **Seizures** originate in the cerebrum and are caused by unsystematic neurologic changes in brain function.
- Seizures are the symptom of an underlying condition.
- Patients may demonstrate convulsive movements or lapse into unconsciousness.
- **Convulsive movements** are categorized as activity in the muscles that is sudden, violent, and uncontrollable.
- **Unconscious patients** or patients with lowered consciousness are usually unable to relate to their surroundings because of a disruption in function between brain hemispheres and the reticular activation system.

- Levels of consciousness are evaluated using the **Glasgow Coma Scale.**

GLASGOW COMA SCALE: Neurologic Portion

Eye response		
Spontaneous	4	
To speech	3	
To pain	2	
No response	1	
Verbal response		
Oriented	5	
Confused	4	
Inappropriate verbalization	3	
Unintelligible verbalization	2	
No response	1	
Motor response		
Follows commands	6	
Localizes pain	5	
Withdraws from pain	4	
Atypical flexion	3	
Extension	2	
No response	1	
Highest possible score		15

- **Manifestations** of seizure may include any combination of the following:
  Jerking, tapping, or rubbing movements
  Flutter of eyelids
  Facial jerking
  Loss of motor activity
  Blank facial expression
  Tachypnea, apnea, or difficulty breathing
  Confusion.

- There are **three types** of seizure:
  Partial or focal
  Petit mal or absence of seizure
  Grand mal or tonic-clonic.

- **Partial or focal seizures** may be either complex or simple.

- During a **simple partial seizure** the patient may retain consciousness.

- A **complex partial seizure** usually begins in the distal portion of an extremity, and the patient suffers loss of consciousness and becomes confused following the seizure.

- **Petit mal** or absence of seizure, usually occurring more often in children, are very brief in duration and difficult to treat.

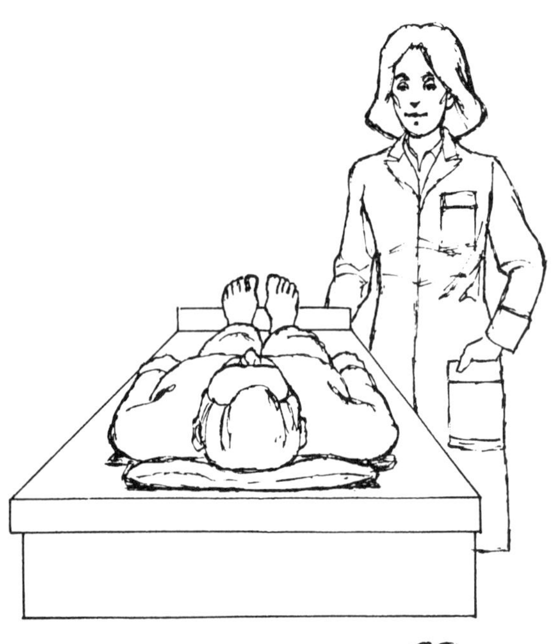

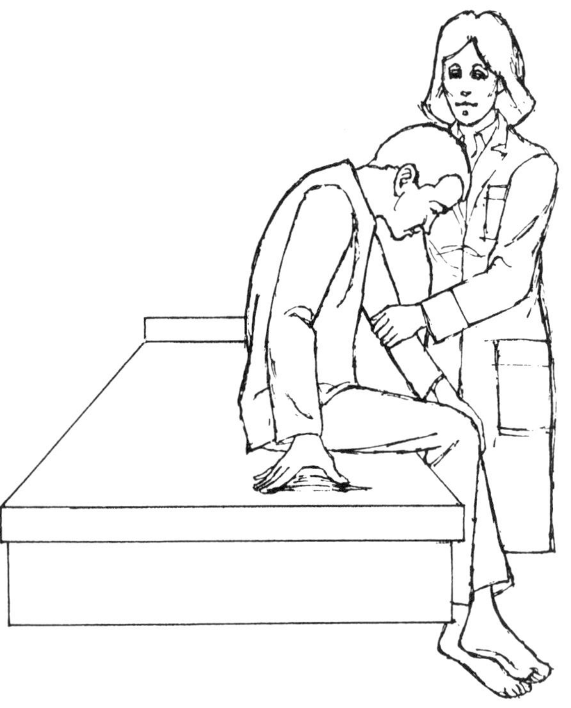

- **Symptoms** of a petit mal seizure include sudden loss of consciousness, eye flutter with obvious loss of focus, and a blank expression.
- A **grand mal seizure** is very obvious in that the entire body usually convulses and the patient experiences a measurable duration of unconsciousness.
- **Symptoms** of a grand mal seizure include muscle rigidity, convulsions, vomiting, incontinence, wide-open eyes, and irregular respiration.
- Possible **complications** of a seizure may be aspiration pneumonia, respiratory arrest or distress, and physical trauma.
- **Radiographers** should render the following aid to patients suffering a seizure:
  1. Ease the patient to the floor or into a safe position.
  2. Remove any objects of potential harm.
  3. Loosen any restrictive clothing and provide privacy.
  4. Do not attempt to restrain the patient.
  5. Note the length and severity of the seizure.
  6. Observe the type(s) of symptoms.
  7. Turn the patient or the patient's head side to the side to maintain an airway.
  8. Assess vitals signs after the seizure has subsided.

FAINTING

- **Fainting** or syncope is caused by low or loss of perfusion to the brain.
- **Causes** of fainting may include but are not limited to

  Orthoscopic hypotension
  Arrhythmia
  Vascular stenosis
  Shock
  Poor diet or fatigue
  Inadequate respiration.
- **Orthoscopic hypotension** is caused by a decrease in systolic pressure due to sudden movement from a recumbent to an upright position.
- **Signs and symptoms** of fainting may include dizziness, sweating, and feeling warm or flushed.

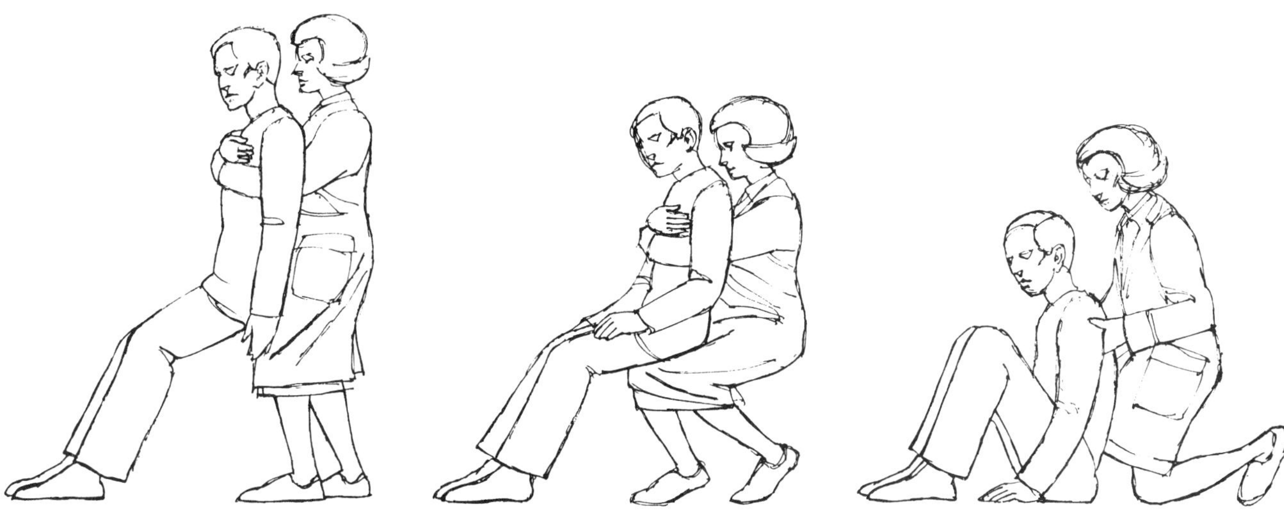

Methods of assistance are as follows:

1. Place your arms around the patient's shoulders and allow him to slouch back toward you.
2. Gently ease the patient to the floor or a wheelchair.
3. Call for assistance as needed.
4. Elevate the legs to increase perfusion to the brain.

SHOCK

- **Shock** results from poor blood flow to the tissues and vital organs.
- There are **four basic types** of shock, categorized by their etiology.
- ***Hypovolemic* or cold shock** can result from either loss of blood volume or plasma volume.
- **Hypovolemia** is the term used to describe a decrease in blood volume.
- **Loss of blood** volume can be caused by trauma resulting in hemorrhage, surgical complications, or gastrointestinal bleeding.
- **Loss of plasma** can occur with dehydration or acute burn injuries.
- **Symptoms** of hypovolemic shock may include
  Syncope or extreme weakness
  Vertigo
  Anxiety or restlessness
  Low and/or falling blood pressure
  Tachycardia
  Tachypnea
  Cool, pale, or cyanotic appearance
  Nausea or vomiting
  Low urinary output.

- ***Vasogenic* or warm shock** is a result of sudden, massive vasodilation.
- As a result of **dilation** of the blood vessels, arterial blood pressure drops swiftly.
- **Vasodilation** may be a result of anaphylaxis, sepsis, or the effects of anesthesia.
- **Symptoms** of vasogenic shock include
  Fainting or dizziness
  Vertigo
  Anxiety or restlessness
  Low blood pressure
  Tachycardia
  Abnormal temperature
  Cool, pale, or cyanotic appearance
  Nausea or vomiting
  Low urinary output.
- ***Anaphylactic* shock** is a type of vasogenic shock due to severe allergic reactions.
- Anaphylactic reactions are caused by the release of histamines in response to foreign substances.
- Common causes of anaphylaxis are insect stings or bites, pollens, and drugs such as penicillin or contrast media administered for imaging studies.
- Anaphylactic reactions or **symptoms** may include
  Wheezing, sneezing, or runny nose
  Hives, edema, or rash
  Nausea and acute vomiting
  Bronchospasm
  Dyspnea and cyanosis
  Falling blood pressure
  Death if left untreated.
- **Cardiogenic shock** is caused by insufficient blood supply to the tissues due to impairment of intravenous function.
- Impairment of **intravenous function** can be a result of acute MI, cardiac surgery, pulmonary emboli, cardiac tamponade, or septal rupture.
- **Tamponade** is a rapid accumulation of fluid in the pericardium which restricts normal cardiac function.
- **Septal rupture** occurs when the septum of the heart ruptures as a result of weakening or trauma.

- **Symptoms** of cardiogenic shock include
  - Altered levels of consciousness
  - Hypotension
  - Anxiety or restlessness
  - Falling blood pressure
  - Tachycardia
  - Chest and/or abdominal pain
  - Ventricular fibrillation
  - Cool, pale, or cyanotic appearance
  - Nausea or vomiting
  - Low urinary output.

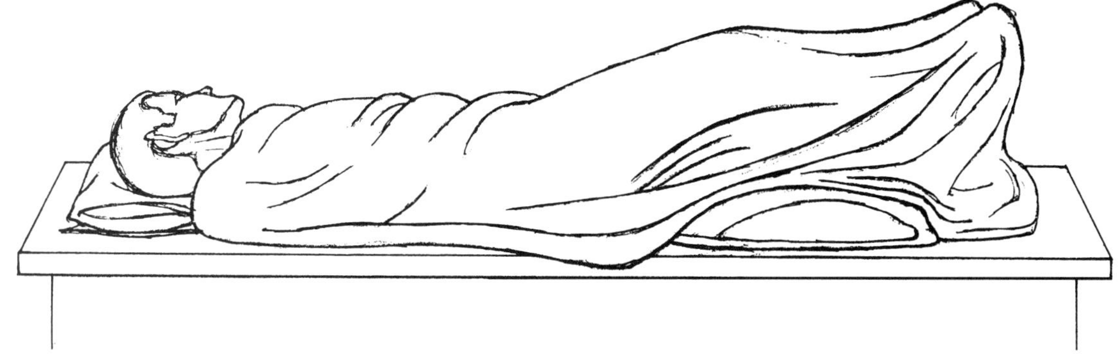

- **Radiographic considerations** involving shock are as follows:
  1. Keep the patient warm.
  2. Elevate the patient's legs provided there are no bleeding wounds in the upper torso or head.
  3. Turn the patient's head or log-roll the patient on her side to prevent aspiration if the patient vomits.
  4. Do not remove extraneous objects for radiographic purposes, such as oxygen or MAST pants (used to redirect blood to vital organs).

DIABETIC EMERGENCIES

- **Diabetes mellitus** is a general disorder caused by improper metabolism and inadequate insulin production.
- **Insulin-dependent diabetes** results in a lack of insulin production, is usually seen in children, and may be genetic. It generally requires the administration of insulin.
- **Non-insulin-dependent diabetes** generally does not require administration of insulin and usually occurs in adults. This condition demands altered dietary habits.

- **Type I diabetes** specifies that autoimmune destruction be present.
- **Type II diabetes** is not characterized by autoimmune involvement.

Comparison of Type I and Type II Diabetes

Characteristic	Type I	Type II
Onset	Abrupt	Gradual
Body weight	Ordinary	Obese
Insulin	Little to none	Some
Control	Insulin and diet	Diet, sometimes insulin
Ability to manage	Difficult	Easy

Comparison of Diabetic Ketoacidosis (DKA) and Hypoglycemia

Characteristic	DKA	Hypoglycemia
Onset	Hours to days	Minutes to hours
Cardiovascular symptoms	Rapid weak pulse, hypotension, warm, dry, flushed skin	Palpitations, pallor, cool, clammy skin
Gastrointestinal symptoms	Abdominal cramps, pain, nausea, vomiting	Hunger, nausea, vomiting
Neurological symptoms	Lethargic, slow reflexes, confusion, coma	Lack of concentration, lack of coordination, anxiety, possible seizures
Respiratory symptoms	Fruity or sweet breath, dyspnea	Increased rate of respiration

- **Gestational diabetes** is a condition occurring during pregnancy in which hormones secreted by the placenta interfere with the action of insulin.
- **Symptoms** of diabetes may include
  Hunger or thirst
  Nausea and headache
  Seeing halos around lights.
- **Hypoglycemia** occurs in persons with diabetes mellitus and is caused by a surplus of insulin in the bloodstream.
- Hypoglycemia may also be **exhibited** by patients who are **fasting** for a specific examination and have taken their insulin but have not had proper food intake.

- **Symptoms** and potential difficulties of hypoglycemia include
  - Headache and nausea
  - Numbness in the extremities
  - Tachycardia
  - Cool, clammy skin
  - Slurred speech
  - Restlessness or anxiety
  - Seizure
  - Shock
  - Possible coma.
- **Diabetic ketoacidosis (DKA)** is a condition resulting from high glucose levels and metabolic acidosis.
- DKA frequently occurs in persons suffering from insulin-dependent diabetes mellitus.
- **Symptoms** and potential problems include
  - Lethargy or slowed reflexes
  - Confusion
  - Sweet or fruity breath
  - Tachypnea
  - Tachycardia
  - Nausea, vomiting, or abdominal pain
  - Shock, renal failure, death.
- **Radiographic emergencies** may occur if the patient is unable to receive insulin because of detainment or extended treatment in the imaging department.
- **Hyperosmolar nonketotic syndrome (HNS)** is a condition in which glucose levels are extremely elevated.
- Causes of HNS may be procedures that require the patient to take nothing by mouth (NPO), prolonged illness, or rehabilitative procedures such as dialysis.
- HNS may also be mistaken for stroke or intoxication because of similar physical manifestations.
- **Symptoms** of hyperosmolar nonketotic syndrome include
  - Confusion, slurred speech, profound thirst
  - Hypotension
  - Dry skin and dehydration
  - Sunken eyes.

Considerations for the Imaging Professional

- Methods of gathering data for the measurement of vital signs should always be documented (rectal versus oral temperature).
- Sites of gathering information for the measurement of vital signs should be documented (radial versus carotid pulse).
- The use of a blood pressure cuff that does not correctly fit the patient's arm may skew the results.
- Imaging personnel should be aware of the proper alert codes and terminology concerning acute care and emergency situations.
- Imaging personnel should be aware of specific patient conditions, such as diabetes, and schedule or modify examinations accordingly.

Chapter 6 Review Questions

1. **If a patient experiences cardiac failure in the imaging department, the radiographer's first course of action should be which of the following?**
   a. Follow emergency protocol and begin CPR immediately.
   b. Rush the patient to the nearest nurse's station.
   c. Leave the room and inform another health care professional.
   d. Begin oxygen administration.
2. **Basic cardiopulmonary resuscitation consists of all but which of the following steps?**
   a. Assess whether the patient's airway is open.
   b. Begin rescue breathing.
   c. Start cardiac compression.
   d. Assess the patient's radial pulse every 10 seconds.
3. **Which of the following results from a clot in the coronary artery (or arteries)?**
   a. trauma to the chest
   b. tachycardia
   c. myocardial infarct
   d. Hypoventilation
4. **Grayish skin tone due to loss of capillary circulation may be caused by which of the following conditions?**
   a. hypoventilation
   b. cyanosis
   c. tachycardia
   d. tachypnea

5. **A clot that loosens and moves throughout the bloodstream is also known as**
   a. a thrombus.
   b. a thromboembolism.
   c. atherosclerosis.
   d. none of the above.

6. **Which of the following is not be a symptom of cardiac arrest?**
   a. cyanosis
   b. tachypnea
   c. seizure
   d. incontinence

7. **Which of the following should be done when caring for a patient with a possible CVA?**
   a. Assess vital signs frequently.
   b. Always have a health care professional attending the patient.
   c. Carefully evaluate the patient's mental state.
   d. All of the above.

8. **Each of the following can be a cause of pulmonary embolism except**
   a. surgery.
   b. trauma.
   c. smoking.
   d. CVA.

9. **Levels of consciousness are evaluated using which of the following scales?**
   a. Mallow's hierarchy
   b. Glasgow Coma Scale
   c. Villate's consciousness indicator
   d. magnetic resonance imaging

10. **Which type of seizure is more likely to occur in children?**
    a. petit mal
    b. complex partial
    c. grand mal
    d. simple partial

11. **Possible complications of a seizure may include which of the following?**
    a. aspiration
    b. physical trauma
    c. respiratory distress
    d. all of the above

12. **If a patient looks as if she is fainting, the imaging professional should do which of the following?**
    a. Assess the patient's vital signs.
    b. Assist the patient to a safe position.
    c. Prepare the emergency cart.
    d. Administer oxygen immediately.

13. **Each of the following could be a sign that a patient may faint except**
    a. sweating.
    b. hunger.
    c. dizziness.
    d. feeling warm.

14. **Orthoscopic hypotension is a condition due to a decrease in ______ caused by sudden movement from a recumbent to an upright position.**
    a. pulse rate
    b. diastolic pressure
    c. systolic pressure
    d. respirations

15. **Generally, a patient showing symptoms of shock has which type of pulse rate?**
    a. rapid
    b. slow
    c. weak
    d. strong

16. **The type of shock caused by a severe allergic reaction, possibly to radiographic contrast, is which of the following?**
    a. hypovolemic
    b. cardiac
    c. septic
    d. anaphylactic

17. **Acute burn injuries, massive blood loss, or uncontrolled gastrointestinal bleeding can result in which type of shock?**
    a. hypovolemic
    b. cardiac
    c. septic
    d. anaphylactic

18. **Which type of diabetes is most common in children and may be genetic?**
    a. gestational diabetes
    b. non-insulin dependent diabetes
    c. insulin-dependent diabetes
    d. hypoglycemia

19. **If a person has a surplus of insulin in his bloodstream, he may suffer from which of the following conditions?**
    a. type I diabetes
    b. type II diabetes
    c. hypoglycemia
    d. hyperglycemia

20. **If left untreated, hyperglycemia may lead to which of the following acute conditions in persons suffering from diabetes mellitus?**
    a. diabetic ketoacidosis
    b. hypoglycemia
    c. hyperosmolar nonketotic syndrome
    d. gestational diabetes

CHAPTER 7

Special Care Situations

CARE OF THE AGING PATIENT

- **Aging** is nonuniform and does not progress at a given rate for every patient.
- **Disease** processes should not be associated with the aging process.
- **Older adults** are classified as being between the ages of 65 and 75.
- **Elder-older adults** are patients over 75 years of age.
- There are changes in the aging patient's physical, sensory, emotional status, etc., which may affect the way in which care should be given.
- **Common changes** due to aging include
  - Decreased vision and hearing ability
  - Difficulty in swallowing
  - Decreased circulation
  - Decreased muscle mass and osteoporosis
  - Decreased sense of smell
  - Diminished ability for quick movement.

Considerations for the Imaging Professional

- The RT has a responsibility to note and observe these changes in order to provide optimum care.
- Give clear directions to the patient and ensure understanding.
- Modify methods of positioning or movement if needed.
- Evaluate the patient for mobility in order to ensure patient safety.
- Provide alternative means, whether written, oral, or nonverbal, of communication to effectively convey directions and describe methods of treatment.

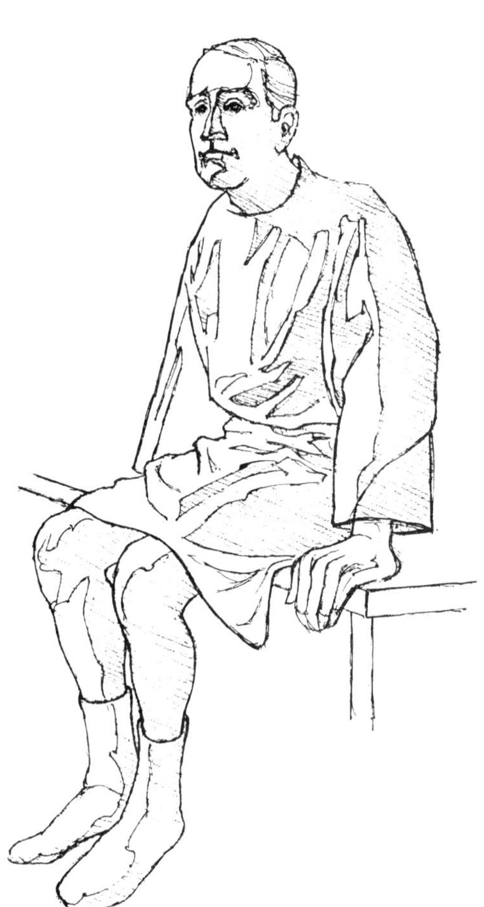

PATIENTS WITH VARIED PSYCHOLOGICAL ABILITIES

- A patient's mental status may be altered as the result of knowledge deficit, an altered thought process, or disorientation .
- **Knowledge deficit** is defined as lacking specific knowledge.
- **Factors affecting knowledge deficit** include lack of exposure, limited cognitive ability, misinterpretation, unfamiliarity, or unwillingness to learn or understand.
- Patients with a deficit of knowledge about the specific examination or situation may exhibit some of the following characteristics:
  - Inability to follow instructions
  - Improper behavior (hysteria, hostility, agitation)
  - Verbalization of their inability to understand
  - Request information to aid in understanding.
- **Altered thought process** is caused by a disturbance in cognitive performance and activity.
- **Factors** that may cause altered thought process include severe sleep deprivation, physiological or psychological changes, and memory loss.
- Some of the following **characteristics** may be exhibited by these patients:
  - Impaired ability to reason and make decisions
  - Obsessions or phobias
  - Delusional or paranoid behavior
  - Inability to follow directions
  - Hyper- or hypoactivity
  - Inappropriate social behavior
  - Hallucinations.
- **Disorientation** is characterized by a patient's inability to identify themselves in relation to time or place.
- Factors that may cause disorientation can be either reversible or irreversible.
- Some causes of **reversible disorientation** are fever, intoxication, electrolytic imbalances, head trauma, and toxic reactions.
- **Irreversible disorientation** may be caused by such conditions as acquired immunodeficiency syndrome (AIDS), dementia, Alzheimer's disease, progressive neurologic conditions, or brain neoplasms.

Considerations for the Imaging Professional

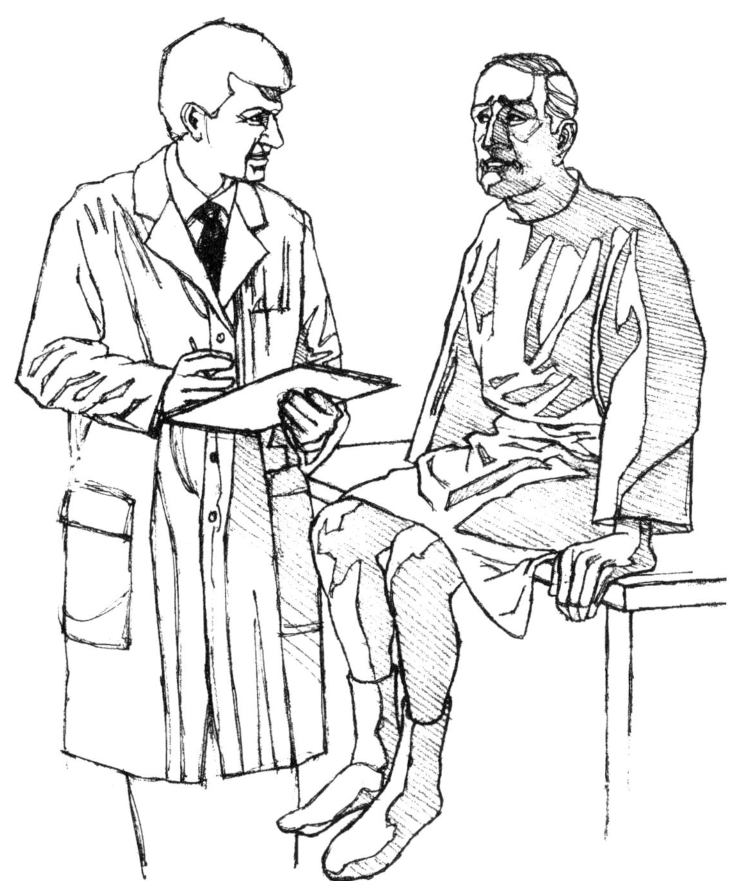

- The technologist should always be alert to patients with a varied psychological status.
- Always encourage conversation and address the patient by name.
- Never point out or mock a patient's behavior(s).
- Whenever possible, contribute positive reinforcement in conversations.
- Be certain that the patient be protected from injury.
- Restraints may be needed for the safe completion of examinations.
- Give simple, precise directions that can be easily understood.
- Alterations in positioning or examination may be required with some patients.

NEEDS OF THE PEDIATRIC PATIENT

- The following are **classifications** of pediatric patients according to age:
  Neonate: child less than 28 days old
  Infant: child between the age of 28 days and 1 year
  Toddler: child between 1 and 3 years old
  Preschooler: child between 3 and 6 years old
  School-aged: child usually between 6 and 12 years old
  Adolescent: young adult 13 to 18 years old
- Each age group within the realm of pediatrics requires different methods of care mainly because of different levels of development.

Neonatal Patients

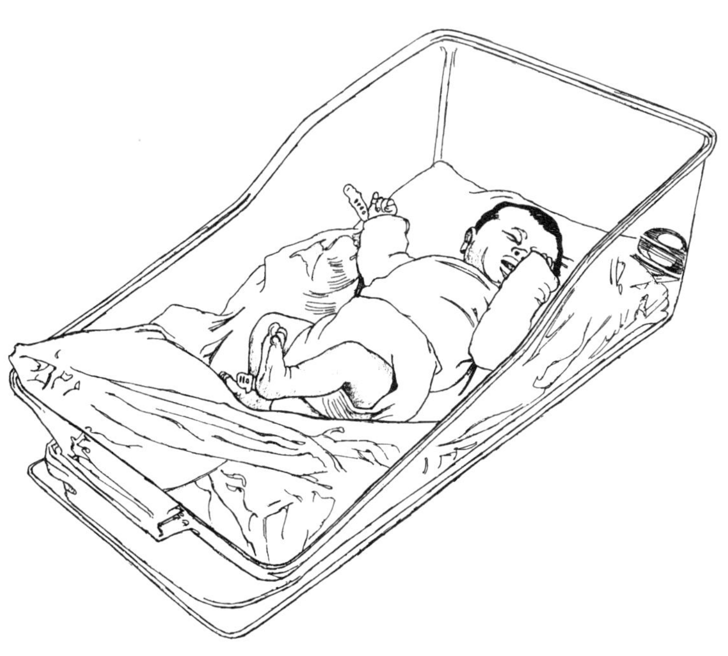

- Most radiographers, unless at a pediatric institution, radiograph neonates in the neonatal intensive care unit (**NICU**).
- Medical asepsis or reverse isolation **precautions** should be employed in the NICU because of the compromised immune systems of the patients.
- Radiographic film, accessories, and portable equipment should be cleaned before entering the NICU.

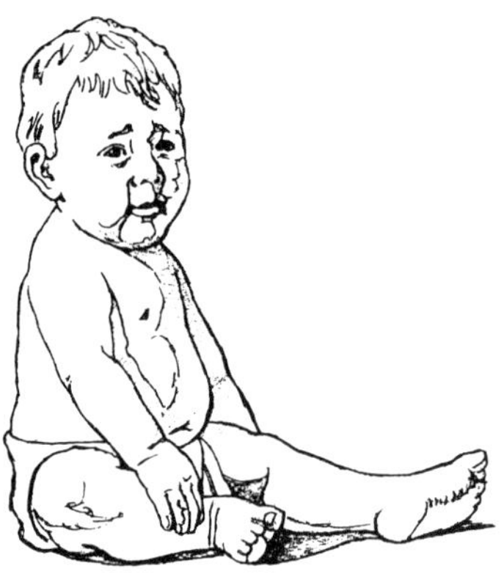

- Strict hand-washing procedures should be utilized.
- It is important that the radiographer obtain detailed information regarding the specific purpose of the radiograph (line placement, respiratory status, etc.) to **avoid repeat examinations.**
- The film should be covered with a sheet or pillowcase in order to prevent direct contact with the patient.
- The radiographer should consult with and request assistance from the nursing personnel before moving the patient to obtain a radiograph.

Infant and Toddler Patients

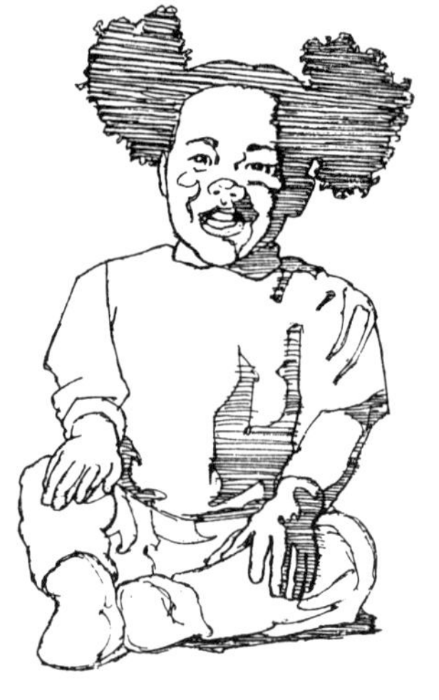

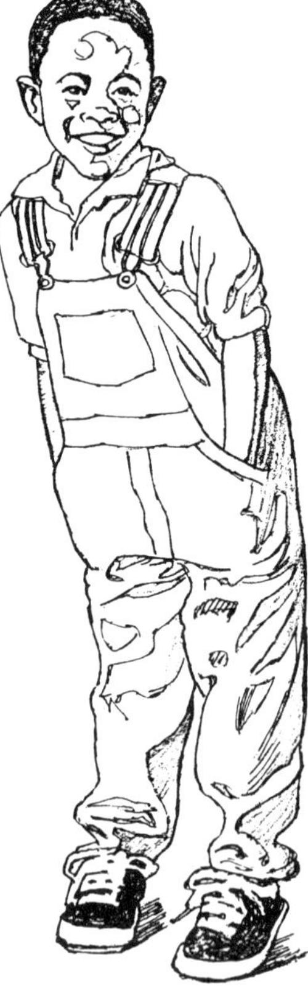

- Imaging professionals may want to **obtain assistance** from the parent(s) in order to reduce stress to the child during the procedure.
- Careful use of **immobilization devices**, such as a papoose board or a Pig-O-Stat, should be utilized.
- Holding patients to immobilize them results in unnecessary exposure and should not be practiced by the imaging professional.
- If it becomes necessary, the parent should hold the child and both should be provided with lead aprons to reduce exposure.
- **A child should never be left alone in the room or in an immobilization device.**
- **Proper technical** factors should be recorded and utilized to prevent needless repeat examinations.

Preschool and School-Aged Patients

- The leading cause of injury in school-aged children is motor vehicle accidents.
- The radiographer should survey the situation to determine whether the child requires the presence of an adult during the examination.
- It is important that rapport be established and that the procedure be explained to the patient.

- The radiographer should answer all questions relating to the patient's care in an understandable manner.
- **Directions** should be given in a simple, precise language that the child can understand.
- It may be advantageous to show the child what needs to be done (positioning, moving, etc.).
- Preschoolers are very curious and enjoy exploring. It is extremely important that they never be left alone.
- Proper **technical factors** should be recorded and utilized to prevent needless repeat examinations.

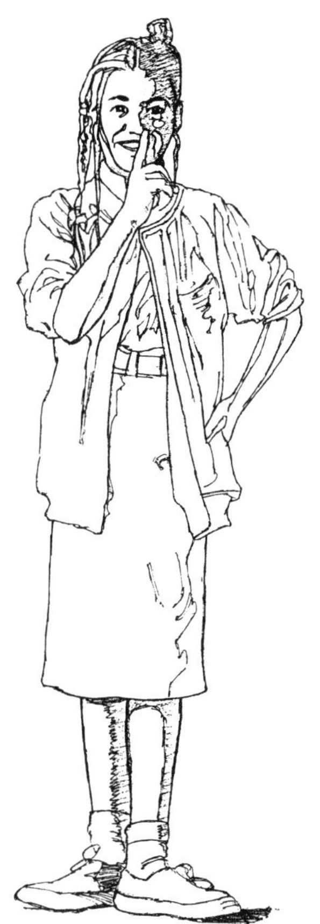

Adolescents

- The leading cause of injury in adolescents is motor vehicle accidents.
- Behaviors that involve alcohol, sex, and drug use may be exhibited at this time.
- It is important to **establish rapport** with the patient and avoid making judgments.
- **Clarify** with the patient any terms or use of language that you may not understand.
- Give clear directions and answer all questions related to the examination.
- Technical factors for the adolescent are usually similar to those used for adults.

Considerations for the Imaging Professional

- The radiographer should assess each situation separately to determine the need for parental involvement.
- Restraints may be needed for safe completion of exams. Patients should not be held.
- Radiographers should give simple, precise directions that can be easily understood.
- Changes in positioning or in the examination may be required with some patients.
- Technique charts employing factors for infants and children should be readily available to avoid repeated examinations.

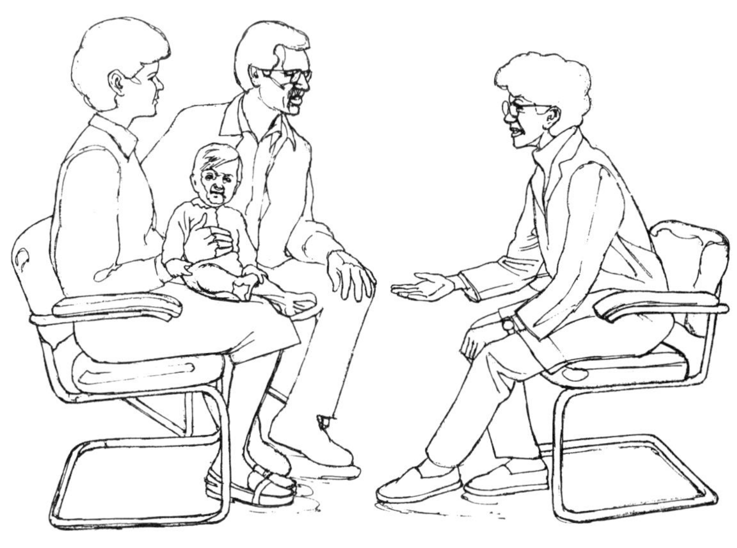

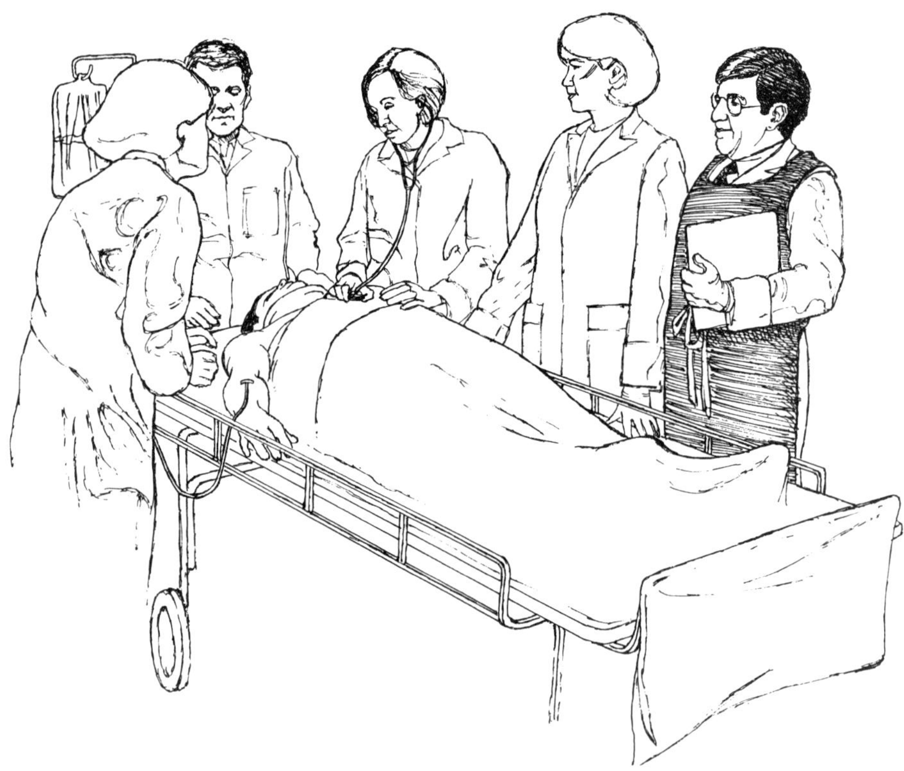

IMAGING THE TRAUMA PATIENT

Emergency Room Examination

- Radiographers have a role on the "trauma team" requiring that quality care be provided in a timely manner.
- The **trauma team** is the group of health care professionals who treat trauma patients in the emergency room.
- It is important that members of the trauma team work together to achieve diagnosis in a short amount of time.

Parameters for Trauma Radiography

- **Prepare** for the specific type of trauma by bringing the proper accessory equipment (grid, film, cassette covers, etc.).
- Advocate that all trauma team members wear aprons.
- **Inquire** of the physician as to the proper method of moving the patient to obtain the radiographs.
- **Communicate** with and solicit the assistance of nurses or physicians when moving patients.

- Do not remove bandages, splints, traction devices, MAST pants, or objects fixed in the patient's anatomy.
- It may be necessary to sacrifice quality in order to obtain radiographs without moving the patient.
- All radiographs should be taken at **90-degree** angles of each other.

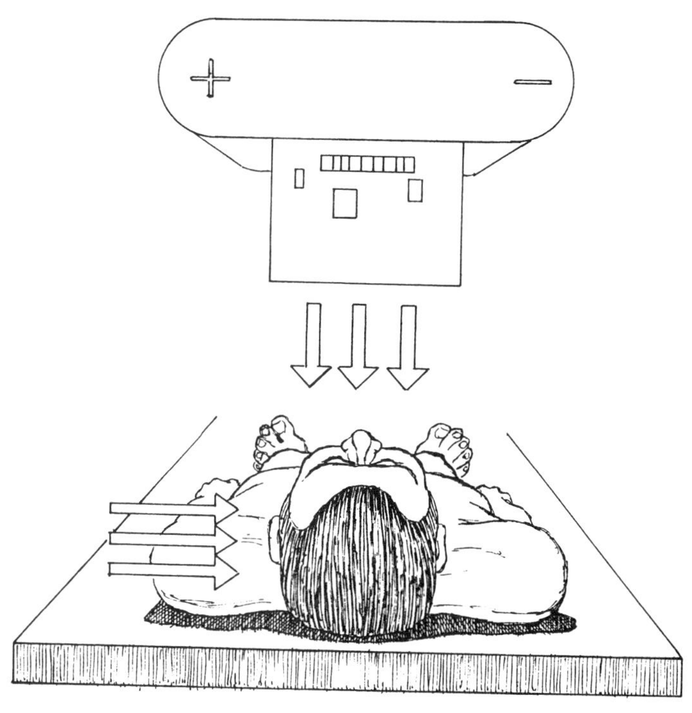

Radiographing Patients with Fractures

Types of Fractures

- **Angulated fractures** are those in which the bone fragments and the factures are at an angle to each other.
- Angulated fractures are usually caused by **direct or lateral force.**
- **Avulsed fractures** involve the pulling away of bone and tissue from ordinary connections.
- Causes of avulsion fractures include direct energy and resisted extension of the area affected.
- **Bucket handle fractures** occur in the pelvis and are double vertical fractures on the same side with a possible vertical fracture on the opposite side.
- Caused by a direct blow or anterior force, these fractures are associated with a dislocation.
- **Closed fractures** are those in which the skin is unbroken in the area of the fracture.
- Closed fractures are generally **produced by lesser force** than other types of fractures.
- **Comminuted fractures** involve the breaking of bones into may pieces. Crushing injuries usually produce comminuted fractures.
- **Compression fractures** are common in the spine and involve condensing of the bone on one side.
- Common causes of compression fracture are axial force applied from above.
- A **greenstick fracture** is manifested by a break on only one side of the cortex and usually occurs in children.

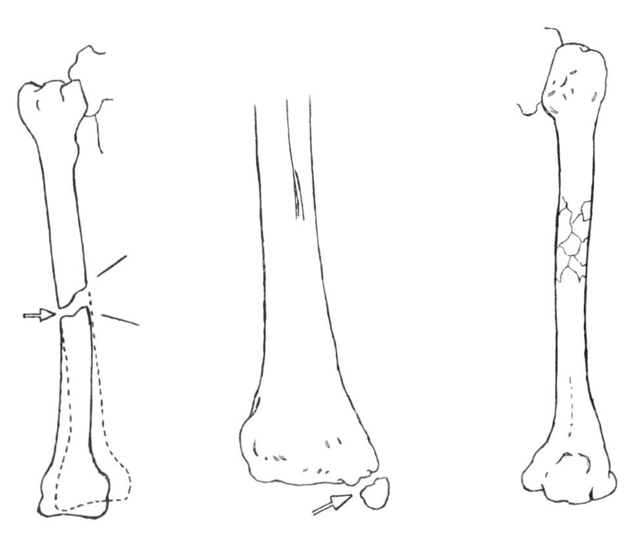

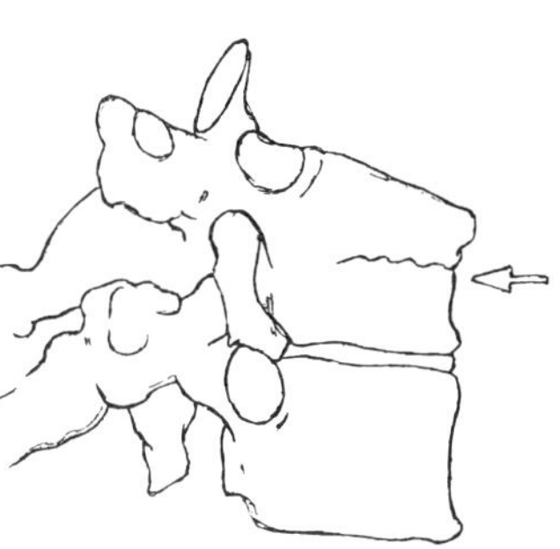

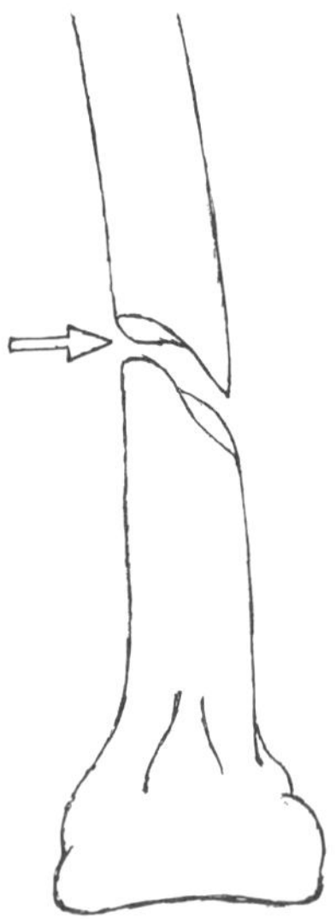

Spiral

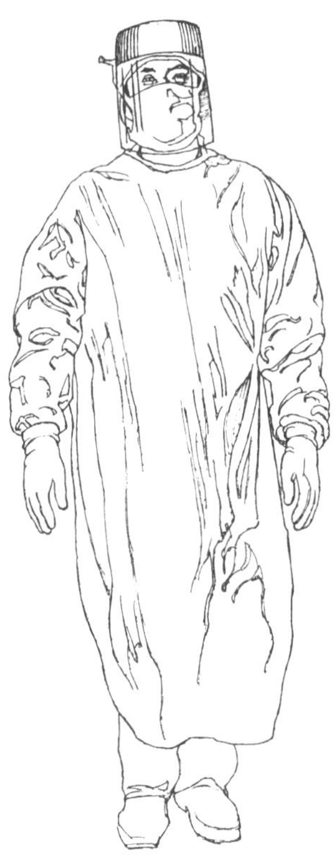

- The cause of greenstick fractures is minor direct or indirect force.
- **Impacted fractures** involve the wedging of bones against each other.
- Impacted fractures are usually caused by axial force distal to the fracture site.
- **Oblique fractures** are angled across the cortex of the entire bone.
- Causes of oblique fractures are compression with direct or indirect force.
- **Open fracture** is the term used to describe the breaking of skin above the fracture site.
- Moderate or extreme force causes the tissue tolerance to be surpassed.
- **Pathologic fractures** may be transverse, oblique, or spiral in nature.
- Pathologic fractures are due to force imposed on bone weakened by tumor.
- **Spiral fractures** curve around the cortex of the bone.
- Spiral fractures are usually caused by twisting of the anatomy when the distal end is unable to move.
- **Straddle fractures** involve the pubic rami and are bilateral.
- Falling with great force directly on an object may cause a straddle fracture
- **Transverse fractures** are crosswise breaks through the bone.

  Direct or indirect force in the direction of the site may cause a transverse fracture.
- **Symptoms** of fractures may include swelling, edema, bleeding, bruising around the site, and shock.
- **Complications** of fractures may involve malunion, nonunion, thrombophlebitis, fat embolism, infection, laceration of an artery, and nerve damage.

Considerations for the Imaging Professional

- Personal protection equipment should be worn at all times. (glove, gown, face shield, etc.)

- The affected part should always be kept immobilized.
- Move the patient under the direction of or with direction from the physician.
- Communicate directions and necessary movement to the patient.
- Cross-table lateral films should be obtained whenever possible.
- When moving the patient, support of fractures should be maintained above and below the fracture site.

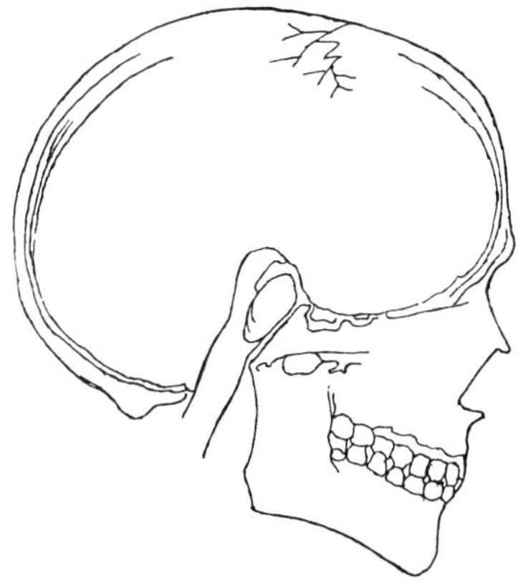

Radiographing Patients with Head Trauma

Skull Fractures

- **Linear fracture** describes a break without bone displacement.
- A **comminuted fracture** consists of multiple breaks with bone fragmentation.
- In a **depressed facture** bone fragments are displaced below the surface of the skull.
- A **compound fracture** is a fracture with laceration to the scalp or membranes.

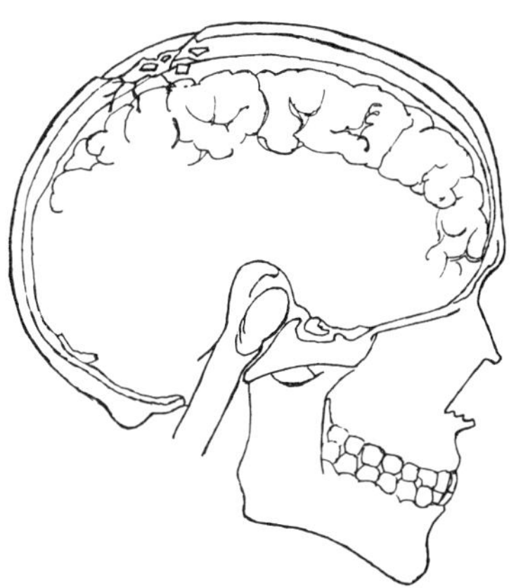

Closed Head Injuries

- A **concussion** is shock to the soft tissue of the brain without bruising or laceration.
- **Symptoms** of a concussion may be memory loss or amnesia (usually only for 48 hours).
- **Contusion** is shock to the brain soft tissue with bruising.
- **Symptoms** include loss of consciousness, amnesia, agitation, stupor, or coma.

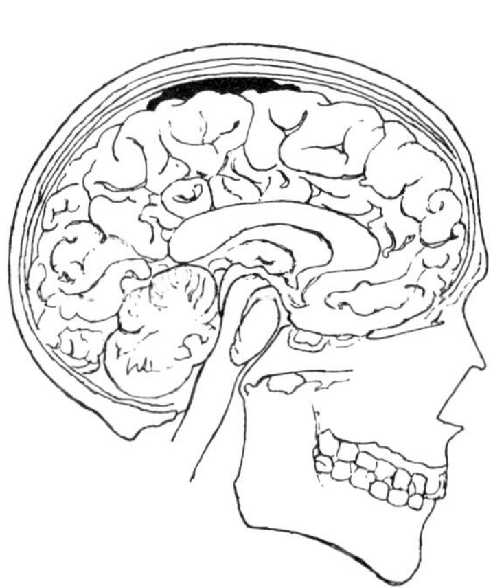

- A **subdural hematoma** is the accumulation of blood between the arachnoid and dura mater resulting from a contusion or laceration of the subdural blood vessels.
- **Symptoms** such as headache, drowsiness, seizure, and unilateral pupil dilation may occur for weeks following a subdural hematoma.
- **Epidural hematomas** involve bleeding into the epidural space between the skull and dura mater.

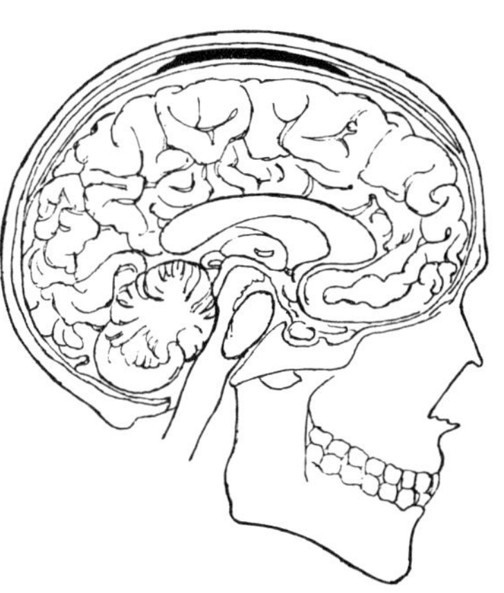

- An epidural hematoma usually involves a **temporal-parietal fracture** that results in a laceration of the middle meningeal artery.
- **Symptoms** include periodic loss of consciousness followed by lucid periods.
- The patient usually has increased **intracranial pressure** (ICP) which requires immediate attention and is a surgical emergency.
- **Complications** of head injuries include
  Increased ICP
  Hemorrhage
  Brain herniation
  Respiratory distress
  Brain damage or deficit.

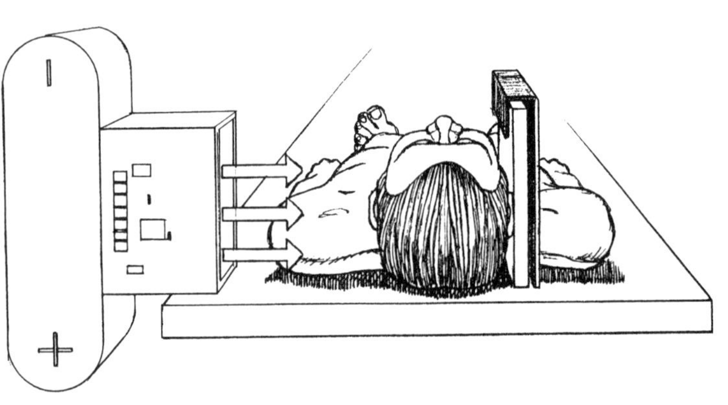

Considerations for the Imaging Professional

- **Personal protection** equipment should be worn at all times (glove, gown, face shield, etc.).
- Skull x-rays should always include a **cross-table** lateral for all trauma head injuries.
- Radiographers should be aware of irregular levels of consciousness or **erratic behaviors.**
- The patient's condition may require **modification** of the examination and/or the assistance to two other people.

Radiographing Patients with Spinal Cord Injuries

- **Cord injuries** result from compression of the cord caused by fracture or displacement of the vertebrae.
- General **manifestations** of cord injury may include
  Loss of power or movement and sensation in extremities below the injury
  Pain at the level of the injury
  Urinary retention.
- **Cervical cord injuries** ordinarily involve levels C2 through C6.
- **Symptoms** of C-spine injuries may include
  Paralysis of all extremities and trunk
  Respiratory failure
  Incontinence
  Sweating, brachycardia, headache
  Neurogenic shock
  Increased temperature.

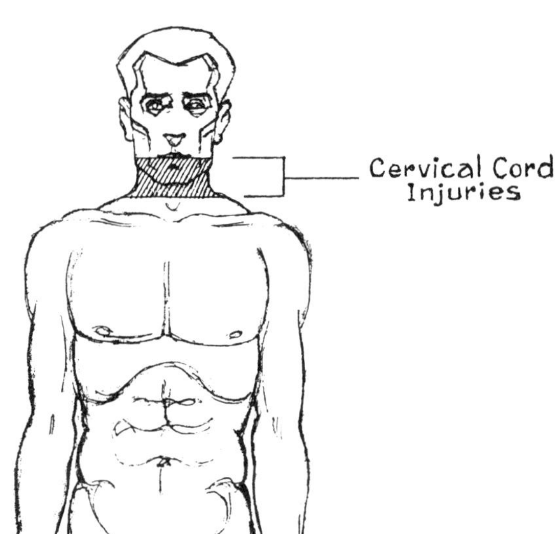

- **Thoracic cord injuries** involve the T1 through T12 vertebrae.
- **Symptoms** of T-spine injuries may include
  Paralysis of the lower extremities
  Flaccid and then rigid muscles
  Paralysis of all bladder and rectal sphincters
  Distended abdomen
  Loss of sexual function.
- **Lumbar cord injuries** usually involve the L1 through L2 vertebrae.
- **Symptoms** of L-spine injuries may include
  Paralysis of the lower extremities
  Loss of bladder and rectum tone
  Flaccid muscles which later become spastic
  Loss of sexual function.

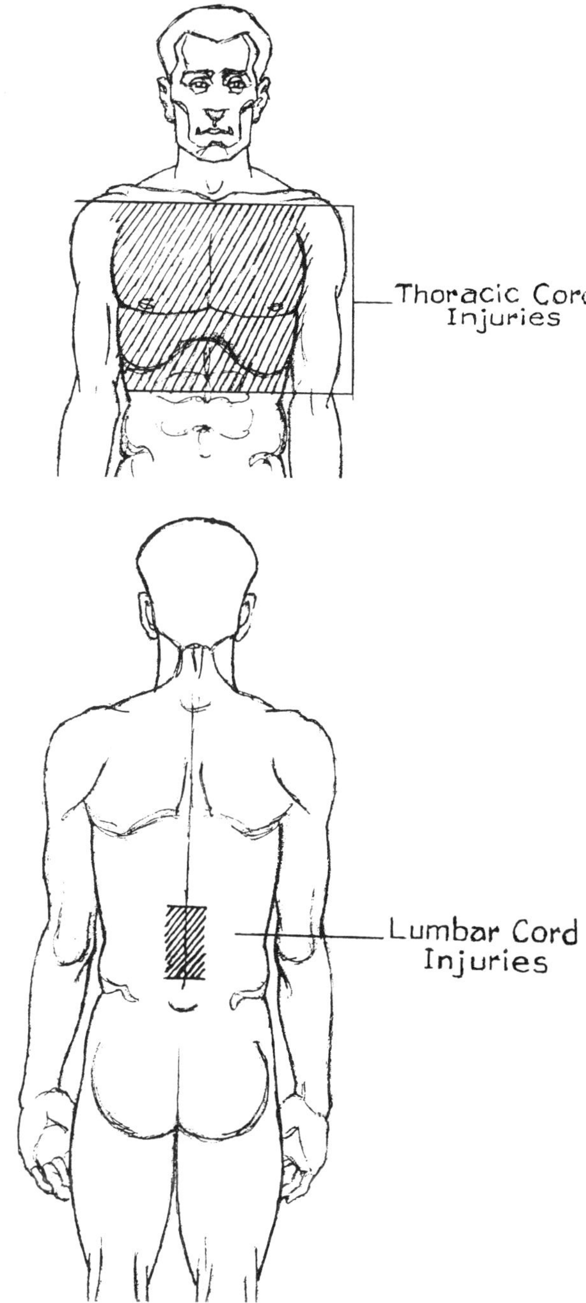

Considerations for the Imaging Professional

- **Personal protection** equipment should be worn at all times (glove, gown, face shield, etc.).
- The patient's condition may require modification of the examination and/or the assistance of two other people.
- Lateral spinal films should be obtained with a cross-table whenever possible.
- Methods of **movement** should be discussed with the physician.
- The patient should not be **log-rolled** without assistance or without the physician's permission.
- Once permission to move a patient is given by the physician, patients with possible cord injuries should **always** be log-rolled.

Chapter 7 Review Questions

1. **How does the aging process progress for each person?**
   a. uniformly
   b. nonuniformly
   c. at a given rate
   d. quickly

2. **Common changes associated with aging include all but which of the following?**
   a. vision
   b. movement
   c. mental capability
   d. body mass or size

3. **If an elder adult cannot move into or maintain a given position during an imaging exam, which of the following would be the best way to accomplish procedure?**
   a. Use whatever method of restraint is necessary to hold the patient in position.
   b. If possible, modify the position to conform to the limitations of the patient.
   c. Cancel the examination and explain to the ordering physician that the patient cannot cooperate in the procedure.
   d. Do all of the above.

4. **Which of the following may be a manifestation of knowledge deficit?**
   a. following instructions inaccurately
   b. verbalizing an inability to understand
   c. requesting information to aid in understanding the procedure
   d. all of the above

5. **Each of the following except ______ may be a symptom of alteration in thought process.**
   a. hallucinations
   b. inappropriate social behaviors
   c. paranoid behaviors
   d. requesting information to aid in understanding

6. **The term used to identify the inability of a patient to identify themselves with relation to time is which of the following?**
   a. altered thought process
   b. disorientation
   c. knowledge deficit
   d. concussion

7. **The leading cause of injury in adolescence is which of the following?**
   a. disease processes
   b. gunshot wounds
   c. motor vehicle accidents
   d. self-inflicted trauma

8. **Which of following patients can be left alone in a room?**
   a. an adult with a head injury
   b. an elder older adult with dementia
   c. a toddler
   d. an adolescent

9. **When imaging a trauma patient, which of the following personnel should wear a lead apron?**
   a. the imaging professional
   b. the trauma physician
   c. the trauma nurse
   d. all the above

10. It is important in trauma radiography to obtain two radiographs taken at ______ of each other.

a. 45 degrees
b. 90 degrees
c. 180 degrees
d. The angle is not important as long as two projections are taken for each anatomy radiographed.

11. In which of the following fractures is the skin unbroken?

a. open
b. closed
c. compound
d. all of the above

12. Which of the following types of fractures are found most often in the pelvis?

a. angulated
b. compound
c. linear
d. bucket handle

13. A common type of fracture that usually occurs in children is called

a. a greenstick fracture.
b. an oblique fracture.
c. a comminuted fracture.
d. a straddle fracture.

14. When moving a person with a fractured extremity, it is important to maintain support

a. above the fracture site.
b. below the fracture site.
c. both above and below the fracture site.
d. either above or below the fracture site.

15. In which type of skull fracture are bone fragments displaced below the surface of the skull?

a. comminuted
b. compressed
c. linear
d. depressed

16. Shock to the soft tissue of the brain without bruising or laceration is termed

a. a concussion.
b. a contusion.
c. a subdural hematoma.
d. an epidural hematoma.

17. In which type of skull fracture is there an accumulation of blood between the arachnoid space and dura mater?

a. concussion
b. contusion
c. subdural hematoma
d. epidural hematoma

18. **Which of the following is not an acute complication of a head injury?**
    a. increased ICP
    b. brain herniation
    c. incontinence
    d. respiratory distress

19. **All of the following are symptoms of a lumbar cord except**
    a. paralysis of the torso.
    b. loss of sexual function.
    c. loss of bladder and rectal tone.
    d. paralysis of the lower extremities.

20. **Which of the following is most important when radiographing a patient with a possible spinal cord injury?**
    a. discussing the injury with the patient
    b. log rolling the patient with assistance when moving
    c. making sure the patient has a draw sheet under him at all times
    d. all of the above

CHAPTER 8

Methods of Respiratory Care

- **Hypoxemia** is a term used to denote symptoms resulting from a lack of proper amounts of oxygen to body organs.
- The brain, retina, and heart are the most sensitive to changes in oxygen levels.
- Symptoms of early hypoxemia may include irritability and memory lapse.
- Hypoxemia is measured arterially and expressed as arterial oxygen partial pressure, Pa_{O_2}.
- **Hypoxia**, or oxygen deficiency, is treated using different forms of oxygen therapy to correct the oxygen insufficiency.
- The majority of respiratory diseases involve some degree of hypoxia.
- The two basic methods used to **monitor** hypoxia are blood gases and pulse oximetry.
- **Arterial blood** is used in measuring blood gases because it has not undergone metabolic changes.
- Three values are obtained for **arterial blood gas evaluation**: Pa_{O_2} (partial pressure of oxygen), Pa_{CO_2} (partial pressure of carbon dioxide), and pH.
- A **pulse oximeter** is a device that allows constant monitoring of oxygen saturation.
- The device measures the amount of oxygen in hemoglobin (oxyhemoglobin) via a sensor probe.
- The sensor probe contains infrared or red light which is absorbed by the oxyhemoglobin.
- The measured amount of absorption is sent to a microprocessor which calculates and displays the values.

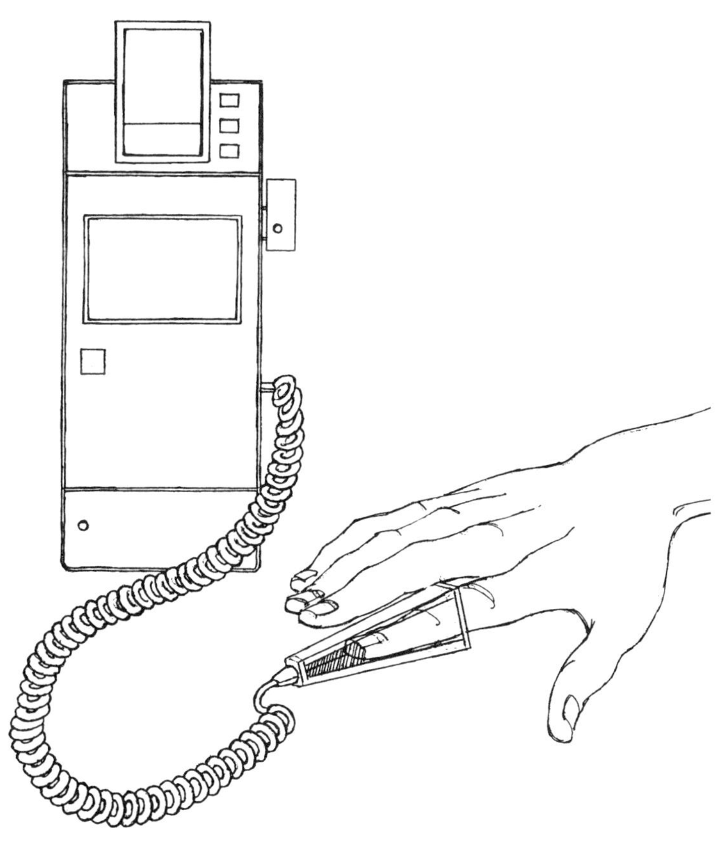

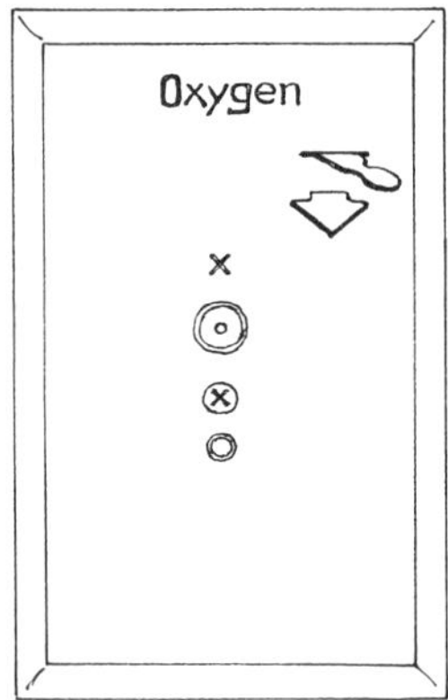

- **Sensor probes** can be placed on the fingertip or on the toe. Adhesive sensors are effectively used on the forehead and nose.

EQUIPMENT FOR OXYGEN THERAPY

- Oxygen is usually obtained in health care facilities by means of a **wall outlet** or a **compressed oxygen tank**.
- Both systems may include a flowmeter, a method for humidifying the oxygen, a length of tubing, and some method of administration.
- The wall outlet may be available throughout rooms in the hospital, including rooms in the imaging department.
- When transporting a patient or if unable to locate a wall outlet, it may be necessary to use an oxygen tank. The tank may contain up to 2000 lb/in.^{2} pressure and should be handled with great care.
- The following **method** should be used when **transferring** a patient from one oxygen source to another to minimize the time the patient is without oxygen.
  1. Check the rate of oxygen flow.
  2. Turn on and adjust the source you will be transferring the patient to before removing the patient from her current source of oxygen.
  3. Remove the patient from her oxygen current source and place her on the new oxygen source as quickly as possible.
  4. Shut off the source the patient is not using.

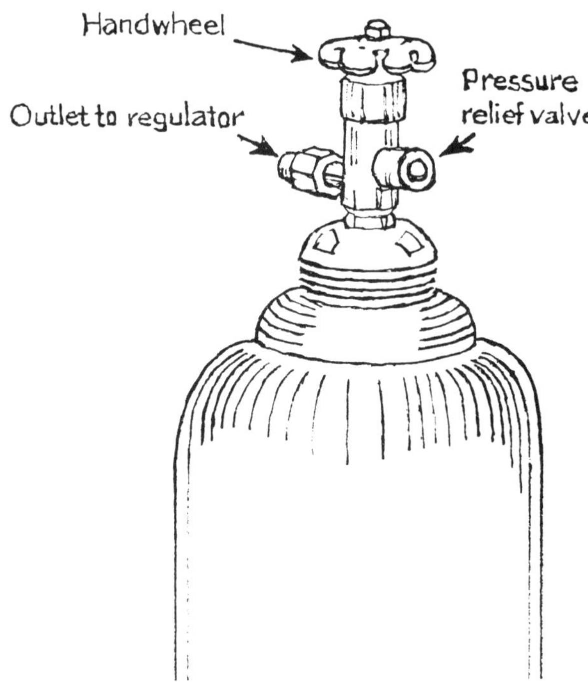

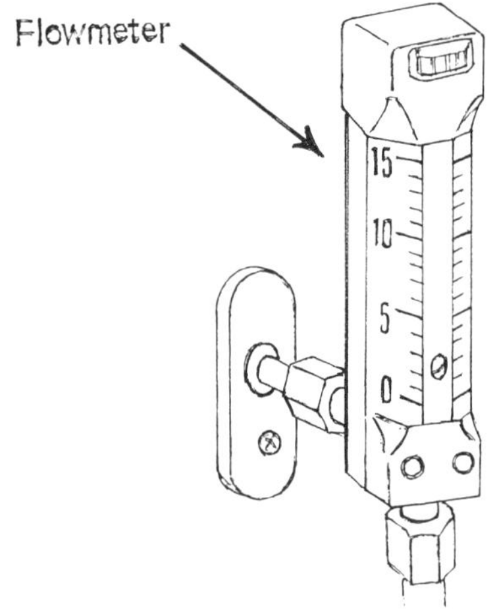

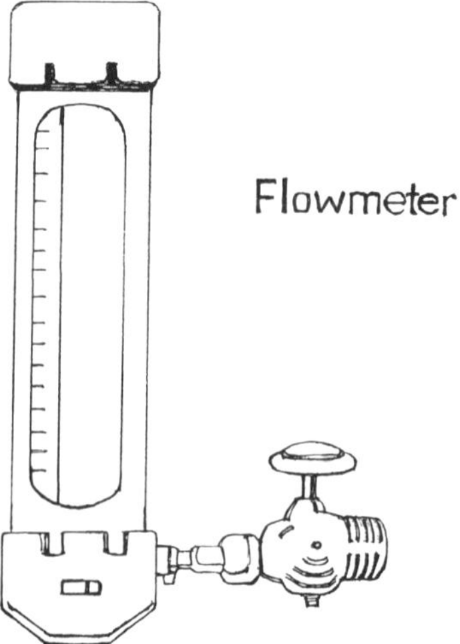

- The radiographer should never place the administration device (nasal cannula, mask, etc.) on the patient and then connect the source of oxygen. This practice may cause great discomfort to the patient.
- **Rates of flow** should always be examined whenever the patient is transported or whenever the source of oxygen has been changed to ensure that proper levels are administered.

STANDARDS OF AIRWAY CONTROL

- The airway is the primary means of ventilation in the human body.
- **Maintaining** an airway and providing oxygen therapy are the most effective treatments for the symptoms of hypoxia.
- Hypoxia is associated with any of the following conditions:
  An obstructed airway
  Anesthesia
  Depressants or drugs
  Respiratory disease processes.
- The brain and heart are the two organs that are the most sensitive to hypoxia and manifest symptoms first.
- When hypoxia occurs, Pa_{CO_2} levels rise, Pa_{O_2} levels fall, and pH falls.
- The lasting **effects** of hypoxia are dysrhythmia and death.

METHODS OF OXYGEN ADMINISTRATION

Nasal Prongs or Nasal Cannula

- **Nasal prongs** or a **nasal cannula** consists of a tube and two prongs (½ inch or less in length) that fit into the patient's nostrils.
- The tubing fits over the ears and is secured under the patient's chin.
- The nasal cannula is **very convenient** as it allows movement and eating with little hindrance.

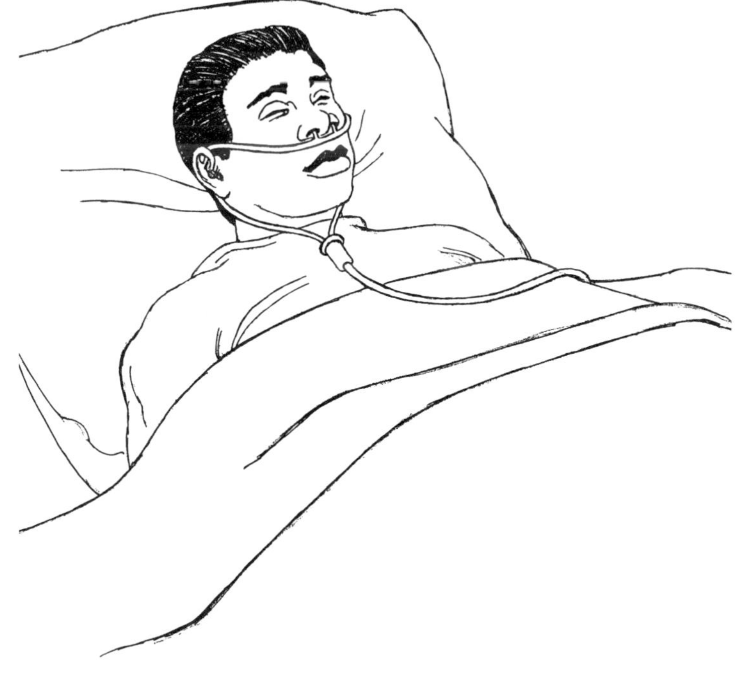

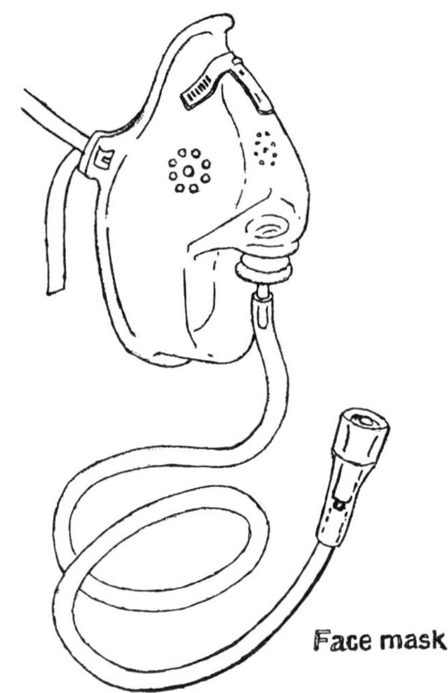
Face mask

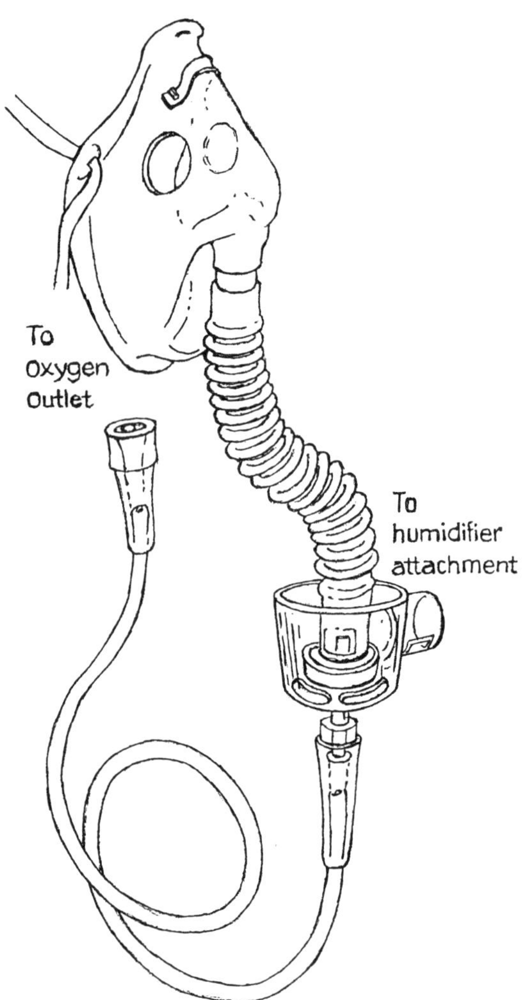

Venturi mask

Nasal Catheter

- A **nasal catheter** is approximately 16 inches in length and is slipped into the trachea via the nose.
- Small holes in the end of the catheter allow oxygen to enter the respiratory tract.
- A nasal catheter is preferred when **high concentrations** of oxygen must be used.
- Like a nasal cannula, the nasal catheter allows for less patient stress, greater mobility, and freedom to continue some normal activities.

Oxygen Mask Systems

- **Masks** are a form of oxygen administration used when the concentration is 25 to 55 percent at flow rates of 3 to 7 L/min (LPM).
- There are several types of oxygen masks, including the face mask, the Venturi mask, the face tent, the nonrebreather mask, and the tracheostomy collar.
- Specific use depends on patient need and the method of administration required.
- A **Venturi mask** is used when a mix of oxygen and room air in precise percentages is required.
- Oxygen can be delivered via the Venturi mask in 24, 28, 35, and 40 percent proportions.
- A **nonrebreather mask** operates using a one-way valve, which controls the flow of exhaled carbon dioxide, and a reservoir bag.
- When the patient inhales, the one-way valve at the reservoir bag opens, allowing only oxygen to be consumed by the patient.
- During expiration, the one-way valve is opened, which allows released carbon dioxide out into the room so as to avoid its accumulation in the reservoir bag.
- A nonrebreather mask delivers 55 to 90 percent oxygen at a rate of 6 to15 L/sec (LPS).
- The rebreather mask does not have a one-way valve and allows carbon dioxide to flow back into the reservoir on expiration.
- A **partial rebreather mask** functions similarly to the nonrebreather system.

- The partial rebreather system delivers 35 to 60 percent oxygen at a rate of 6 to 12 LPM.
- Using a nebulizer, the aerosol mask delivers 35 to 100 percent oxygen mixed with water particles at various rates.
- A **face tent** is a device some patients may find more comfortable, as it does not fit tightly over the nose and mouth but is snugly fitted against the chin.
- Although it may provide greater comfort, this type of mask is less precise with reference to both administration and uptake rates.
- A **tracheostomy collar** is used to provide an oxygen water mist to patients with tracheostomy tubes who require oxygen but do not need a mechanical ventilating device.

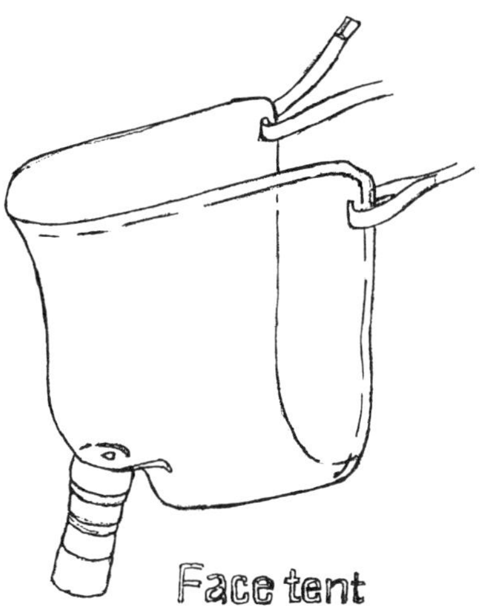

Face tent

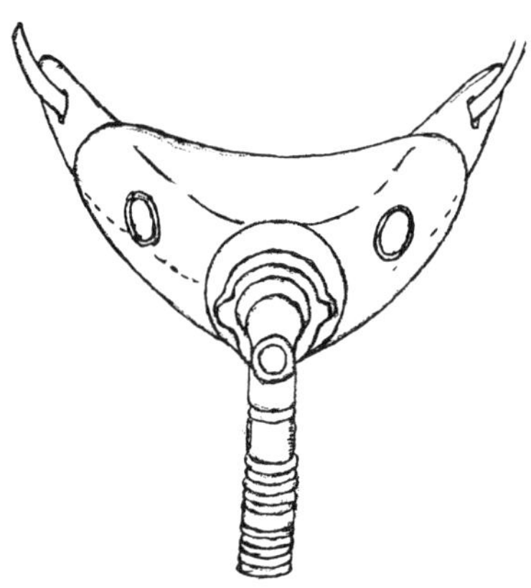

Trach collar

Oxygen Tent

- The purpose of an **oxygen tent** is to provide high concentrations of oxygen and to circulate humidified air.
- The oxygen tent should be opened as little as possible in order to maintain the correct oxygen concentration.

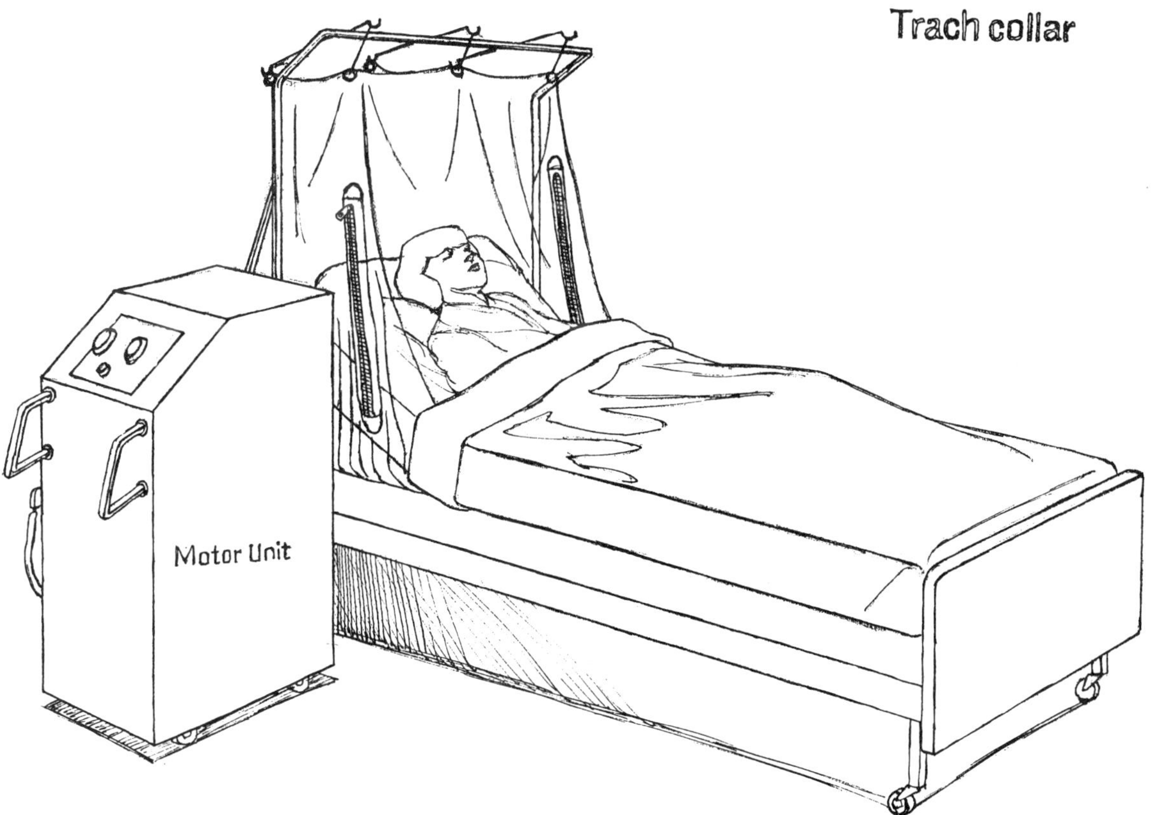

- When performing portable radiography on patients being treated with this system, it may be necessary to shut off the therapy while completing the examination.
- Oxygen tents are most commonly used in pediatric units within the hospital.

Mechanical Ventilation Systems

- **Mechanical ventilation systems** are commonly termed **respirators**.
- A mechanical ventilator is frequently used to provide oxygen therapy for patients unable to breath on their own.
- The **rates regulated** by the mechanical ventilator include the amount of air in each breath, the amount of oxygen supplied, and the rate of respiration.
- The radiographer should be cautious when radiographing patients on mechanical ventilation so as not to dislodge the endotracheal tube.

Considerations for the Imaging Professional

- Oxygen is a gas and may produce lethal effects if not administered correctly.
- Since oxygen is a gas, it is highly combustible. Care should be taken to avoid fire hazards created by the presence of oxygen.
- Infection spreads easily and bacteria flourishes in an oxygenated environment. For this reason contaminated materials should be quickly discarded when treating patients on oxygen therapy.
- Oxygen may dry out mucous membranes and tissues, which also encourages the spread of infection.
- Oxygen tanks should be handled with caution. They should be stored in carriers at all times.
- If a carrier is not available, a tank should be placed on its side for storage or transport and should never be stood upright.
- If an oxygen tank falls and damage to a valve occurs, the tank may become a projectile, causing damage and immense harm.

INTUBATION AND SUCTION PROCEDURES

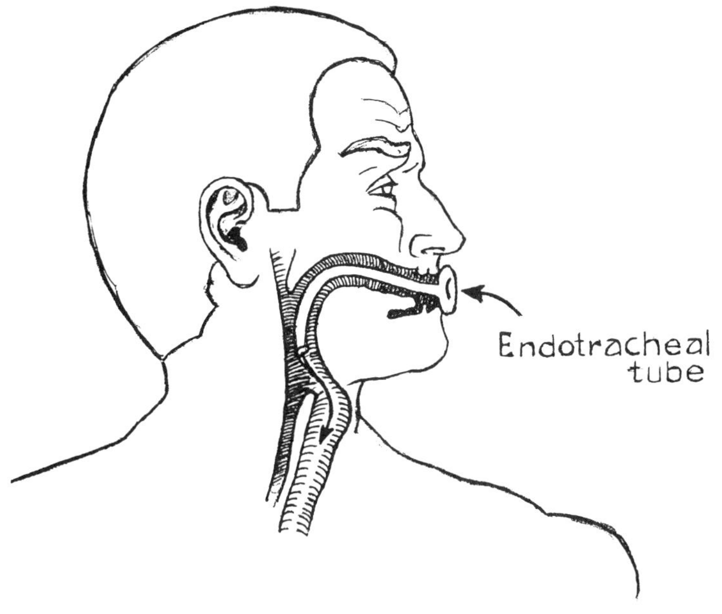

- **Intubation** is the term used to describe insertion of a tube to establish or maintain an airway.
- There are **two types** of pharyngeal airway tubes: the endotracheal tube and the nasal airway tube.
- An **endotracheal tube** is a hollow hard plastic tube that is usually inserted into the patient's mouth during emergency or surgical situations.
- An endotracheal tube acts to maintain an airway and prevents the tongue from falling back into the throat and blocking the process of respiration.
- Similarly, a **nasal airway tube** is inserted into the pharynx via the nose.
- This tube is used to maintain an airway in patients unable to breath on their own.
- The average length of time an endotracheal tube or nasal airway can be used is 5 days.
- Because of mucosal ulcerations, it may be necessary for a **tracheostomy tube** to be inserted if airway maintenance is required for an extended period.
- Tracheostomy tubes are inserted via a small incision or tracheotomy in the neck.
- A tracheostomy tube acts to maintain an airway with the use of an endotracheal tube or tracheostomy tube.
- Tracheostomy tubes may be permanent if the patient's condition requires continued airway maintenance.
- **Suctioning** of tracheostomy and endotracheal tubes is an important part of airway maintenance.
- A need for suctioning of the tubes may be indicated by the patient's respiratory sounds.
- It should be noted that suctioning can interfere with arterial oxygenation and may cause heart dysrhythmias, arrhythmias, and possibly cardiac arrest.

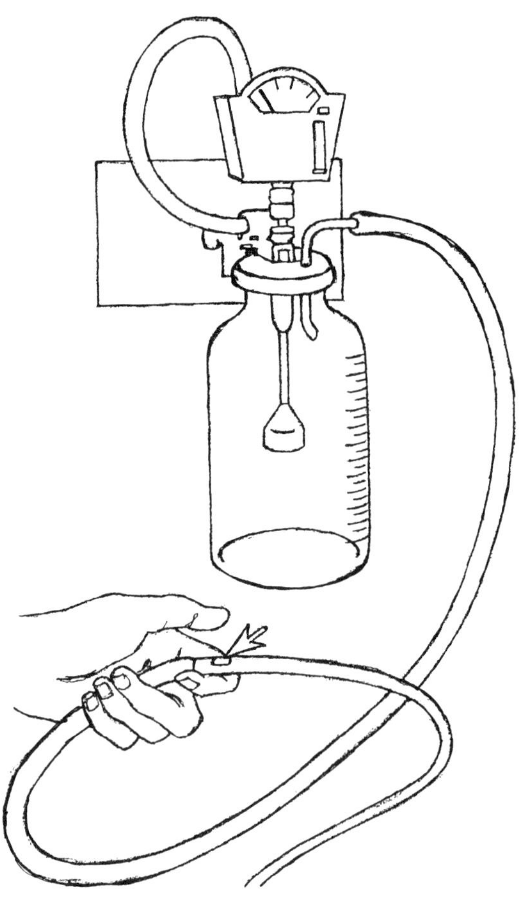

- The **process** of suctioning a patient with a respiratory illness and generally in poor health should be carefully monitored.
- It is common to **oxygenate** most patients before and after suctioning in order to counteract arterial deoxygenation.
- Suction should be used only in patients who cannot discharge secretions by coughing.
- Common suctioning **devices** include the portable electric model and the wall-mounted suction device.
- All suction equipment should be properly disinfected after use. Disposable supplies are currently preferred.

Chapter 8 Review Questions

1. **Which of the following organs is the most sensitive to changes in oxygen levels?**
   a. retina
   b. brain
   c. heart
   d. all of the above
2. **Lack of proper amounts of oxygen may cause which of the following conditions?**
   a. hypoglycemia
   b. hypoxemia
   c. hypotension
   d. anemia
3. **The type of blood used to measure blood gases is which of the following?**
   a. hemoglobin
   b. venous
   c. arterial
   d. all of the above

4. **A pulse oximeter measures**
   a. rate of respirations.
   b. rate of pulse.
   c. amount of blood pressure.
   d. amount of oxygen saturation.

5. **What are the two primary methods of treating hypoxia?**
   a. provide oxygen therapy and maintain an airway
   b. provide intravenous fluids and oxygen therapy
   c. place the patient in the Trendelenburg position
   d. administer medication and provide intravenous fluids

6. **Which method of oxygen administration should be used on an ambulatory patient requiring high concentrations of oxygen?**
   a. nasal prongs
   b. nasal catheter
   c. oxygen tent
   d. mechanical ventilation

7. **Which type of oxygen mask delivers the highest percentage of oxygen at the fastest rate?**
   a. Venturi mask
   b. nonrebreather mask
   c. partial rebreather mask
   d. face tent

8. **What is commonly regulated when using a mechanical breathing system?**
   I. amount of oxygen per breath
   II. amount of oxygen supplied
   III. rate of respirations

   a. I and II
   b. II and III
   c. I and III
   d. I, II, and III

9. **Which of the following is a true statement regarding oxygen?**
   a. Oxygen is a gas.
   b. Oxygen is combustible.
   c. Oxygen may be toxic.
   d. a and b are true.
   e. a, b, and c are all true.

10. **If a patient can breath but an airway cannot be maintained, which of the following can be employed?**
    a. endotracheal tube
    b. nasal airway
    c. tracheostomy tube
    d. suction device

11. When should one suction an endotracheal or tracheostomy tube?

a. at least once a day
b. when secretions can not be discharged and are hindering normal respiration
c. when secretions are visible
d. only when the physician is present

12. Which of the following can occur as a result of suctioning?

I. dysrhythmia
II. arrhythmia
III. deoxygenation
IV. ulcerations

a. I and II
b. II, III, and IV
c. I, II, and III
d. I, II, III, and IV

Gastric, Chest, and Urinary Catheters

CHAPTER 9

NASOGASTRIC, INTESTINAL, AND ENTERAL FEEDING TUBES

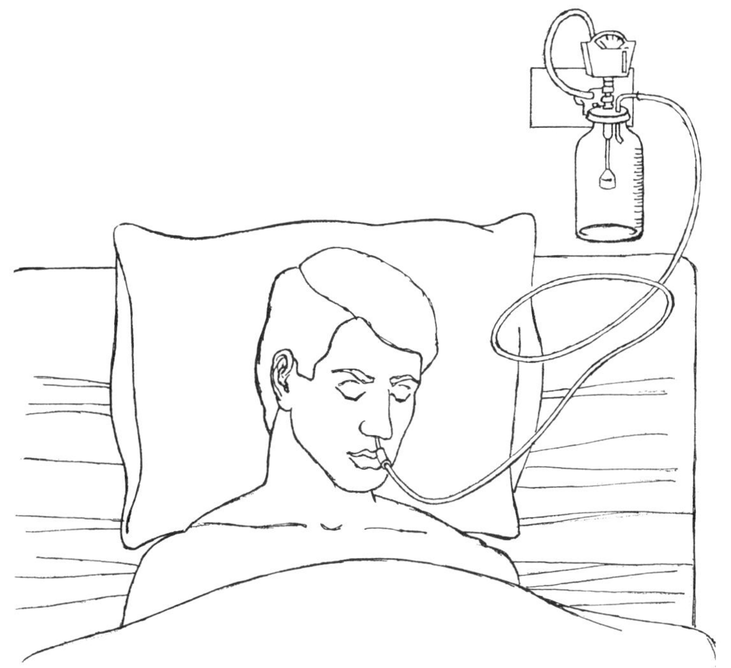

- A **nasogastric (NG) tube** is a tube that is inserted into the nose, through the esophagus, and into the stomach.
- The **primary reasons** for inserting a NG tube are
  - To drain stomach contents.
  - To prevent postoperative vomiting, obstruction, or distention of the GI tract.
  - To acquire stomach secretions in order to diagnosis disease.
  - To flush out ingested toxins.
  - To provide a route for nonoral feeding.
- There are various **types** of GI tubes that serve a similar purpose yet differ in design. The two used most prevalently are the Levin and the sump tubes.
- A **Levin tube** is a rubber or silicone tube which is commonly used for suction, gastric drainage, or stomach feeding.
- A Levin tube is a single-lumen tube which may be up to 36 inches in length and has holes at the distal end.

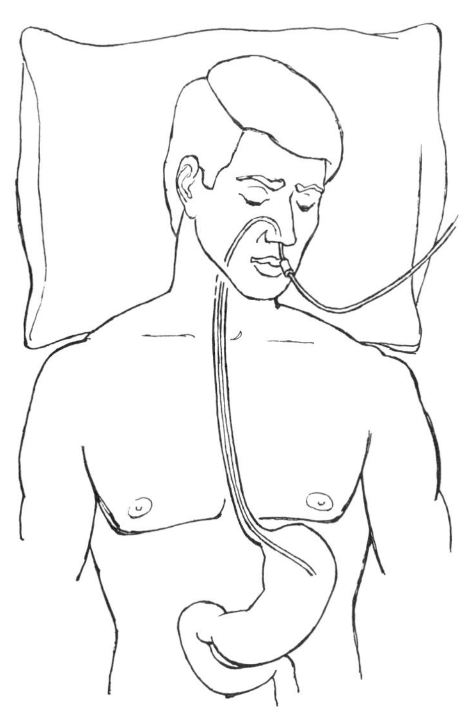

- A **gastric sump** tube is a double-lumen tube which allows emptying of the stomach contents and minimization of the pressure caused by suction.
- The double lumen is located proximally, while the distal tip contains holes similar to those in the Levin tube.
- One lumen is hooked to the suction while the other lumen, or pigtail portion, acts as a ventilation device.
- Other types of gastric sump tubes include the Ventrol, Salem, and Moss tubes.

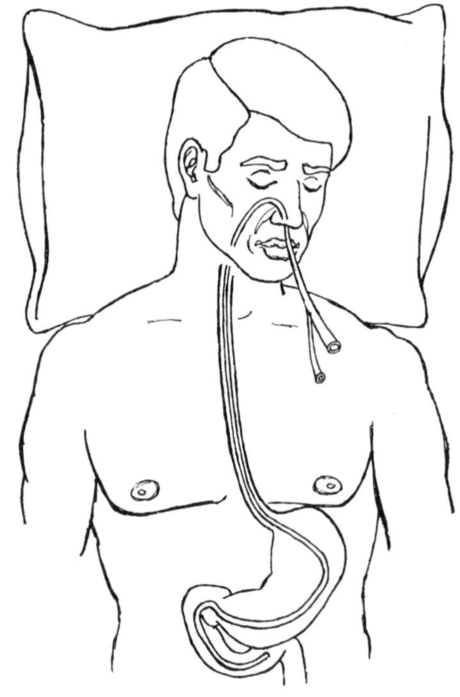

- **Nasoenteric** (NE) **tubes** are inserted through the nose into the esophagus and stomach but usually pass through the stomach into the small intestine.
- Nasoenteric tubes are used to drain contents, analyze secretions, or act as a method for feeding.
- **Nasoenteral tubes** are normally used to feed patients who cannot take in food orally.
- The nasoenteral method of feeding is used most often with patients who have disease processes or conditions such as coma that prevent oral ingestion of food.
- There are various **types** of nasoenteral feeding tubes, including the standard Levin, Keofeed, and Nutriflex tubes and the Dobhoff feeding tube.

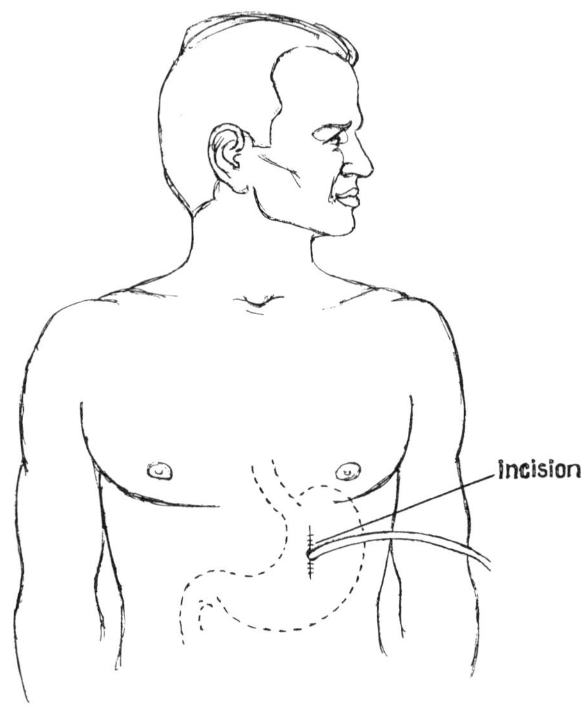

Surgically Placed Feeding Tubes

- **Gastrostomy tubes** are placed surgically or by the percutaneous endoscopic method.
- The tube can be removed and replaced as needed via the healed incision.
- **Jejunostomy tubes** are slipped into the jejunum surgically and permanently sutured into position.
- A jejunostomy tube is used primarily with patients who are at risk for reflux aspiration.
- Jejunostomy and gastrostomy tubes are used to feed patients who cannot feed orally.

Gastric Suction

- Imaging professionals usually are not required to perform gastric suction.
- **Suction machines** secured to a gastric tube act to remove stomach contents by creating low pressure.
- **Low continuous suction is used**, which prevents suction of the gastric tissue into the holes in the distal end of the gastric tube.
- If it is necessary to perform gastric suction, the radiographer should consult the physician or nursing personnel before starting the procedure.

CHEST AND WATER SEAL DRAINAGE TUBES

- The **two layers** of the lungs, the parietal pleura and the visceral pleura, slide against each other during normal respiration.
- Trauma or pathologic conditions may cause there to be too much space between the linings, hindering normal respiration.
- **Common conditions** that cause separation of the space are pneumothorax, hemothorax, and hemopneumothorax.
- A **pneumothorax** is a collection of air in the pleural space caused by pathology or trauma.
- The two basic types of pneumothorax are an open pneumothorax and a closed pneumothorax.
- An **open pneumothorax** is also referred to as a "sucking chest wound" because air is allowed to move in and out of the chest wall through the wound opening.
- A **closed pneumothorax** injury causes air to be trapped in the pleural space, restricting lung expansion.
- Large veins that carry blood to the heart may also be compromised, which may lead to death.
- **Chest tubes** are inserted to help reestablish proper pressure and drain the pleural space.
- The chest tube is inserted through an opening or thoracotomy in the chest wall and placed in the pleural cavity.
- The chest tube is attached to a **water seal drainage system** which allows air to escape the pleural cavity, reducing the pneumothorax, and seals off any air trying to enter the pleural cavity.

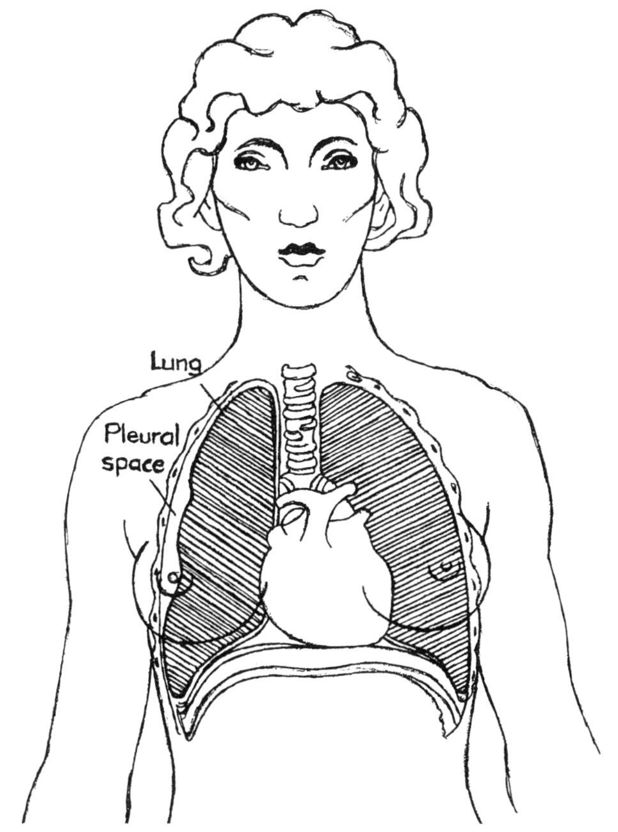

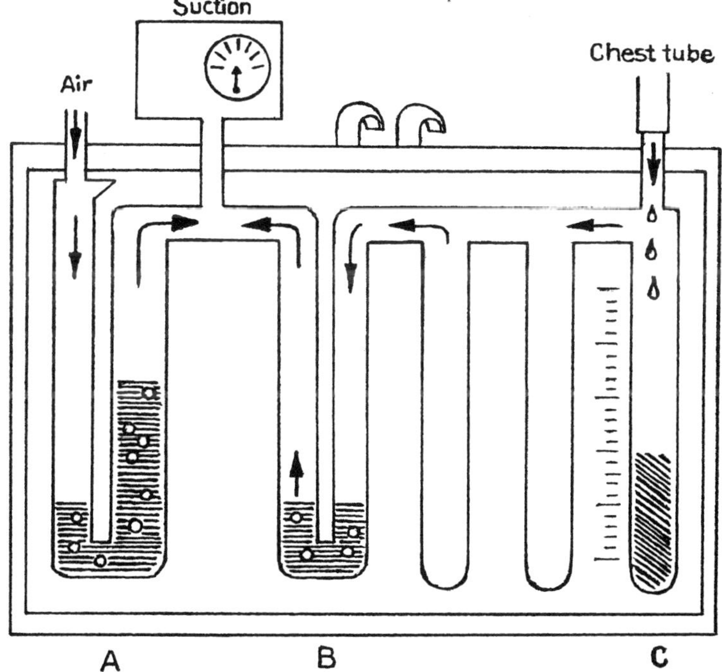

Considerations for the Imaging Professional

- Unless instructed by a physician, chest tubes should not be clamped.
- Avoid disconnection of the tubes and water seal apparatus by ensuring that all connections are secure before moving the patient.

- The water seal should be kept lower than the patient's chest at all times.
- Excess tubing should be secured at the level of the drainage system and not be allowed to hang below the drainage system.
- The water seal system should be kept upright at all times, and contents should never be removed.
- Ensure that the patient has an adequate amount of tubing to allow for movement during radiographic procedures.

URINARY CATHETERIZATION

- It may be necessary for the imaging professional to catheterize patients for such imaging procedures as the cystogram and the voiding cystogram.
- When **performing** urinary catheterization, the imaging professional should use medical aseptic techniques.
- The urinary bladder is **sterile**, and urinary catheterization is a sterile procedure.
- **Catheterization** may be required for any of the following reasons:
  - To alleviate bladder distention when a patient cannot void
  - To obtain a specimen for analysis
  - In preparation for a surgical procedure
  - To drain the bladder of a patient with chronic incontinence
  - As a means of urine measurement
  - As a route to administer contrast for an imaging procedure.
- Various types of catheters can be employed depending on the reason for the procedure.
- A **straight catheter** is most often used to obtain a specimen or drain the bladder.
- A **Foley catheter** is the most common type available for extended use.
- A Foley catheter is a double-lumen tube which allows inflation of a small balloon to hold the catheter in the bladder. The second track allows urinary drainage.

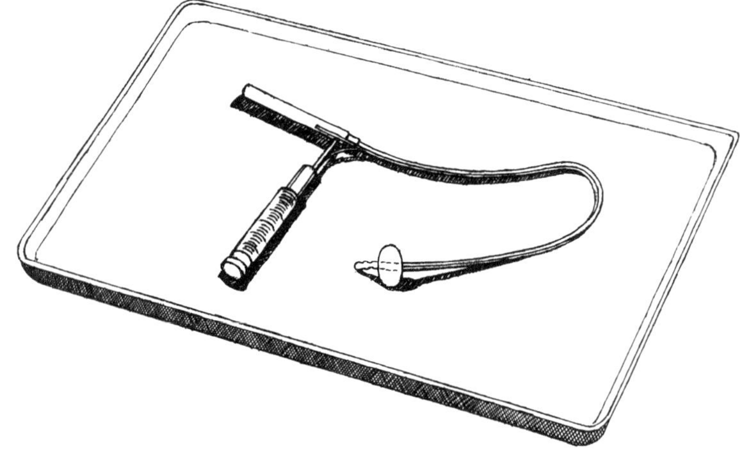

- It is important to note that approximately 5 to 10 ml of sterile water is used to inflate the balloon and must be removed before attempting to remove the catheter.
- A common triple-lumen catheter is the **Alcock catheter.** One lumen provides drainage, another provides inflation of the balloon, and the third provides a site for infusing irrigation.

Female Catheterization

- When catheterizing a female patient **sterile supplies** and **aseptic technique** must be used.
- Proper hand washing, gloving, and surgical asepsis should be employed. It is also necessary to prepare and attach the syringe containing sterile water before beginning to cleanse the area.
- The patient should be placed in the **lithotomy** position in order to cleanse the meatus with the aseptic solution contained in the catheterization kit.

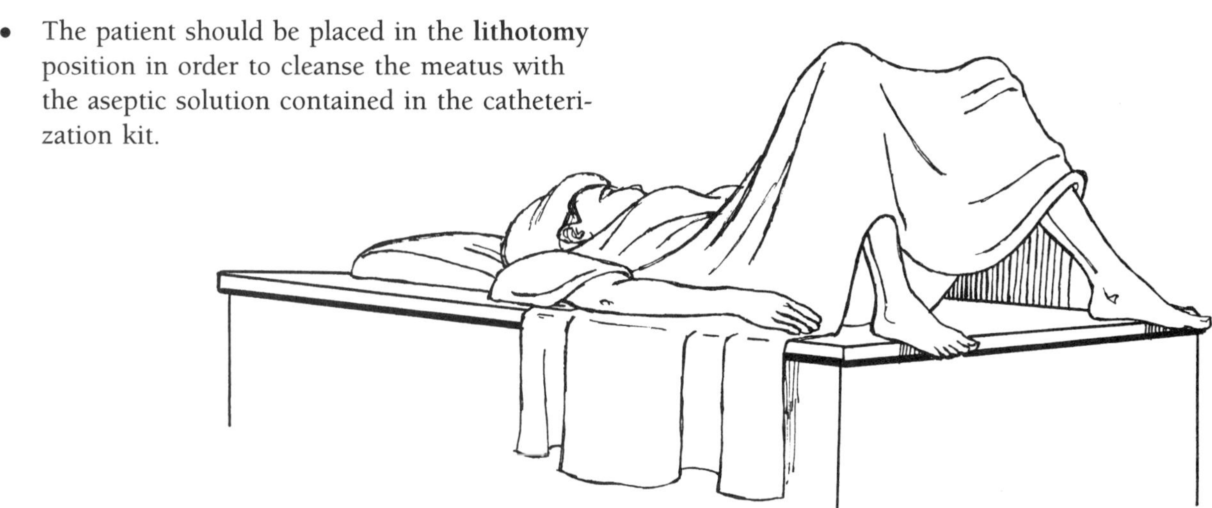

- It is necessary to **cleanse** the area thoroughly, cleaning the distal, proximal, and central portions of the area.
- With the tip of the catheter lubricated, **insert** the catheter into the meatus.
- The female urethra is usually 3 to 5 cm in length. The bladder is reached when urine begins to flow through the catheter.
- **Advance** the catheter at least 2 cm further and inflate the balloon with sterile water in order to secure the catheter.
- It is important to tape the catheter to the leg in order to ensure security.

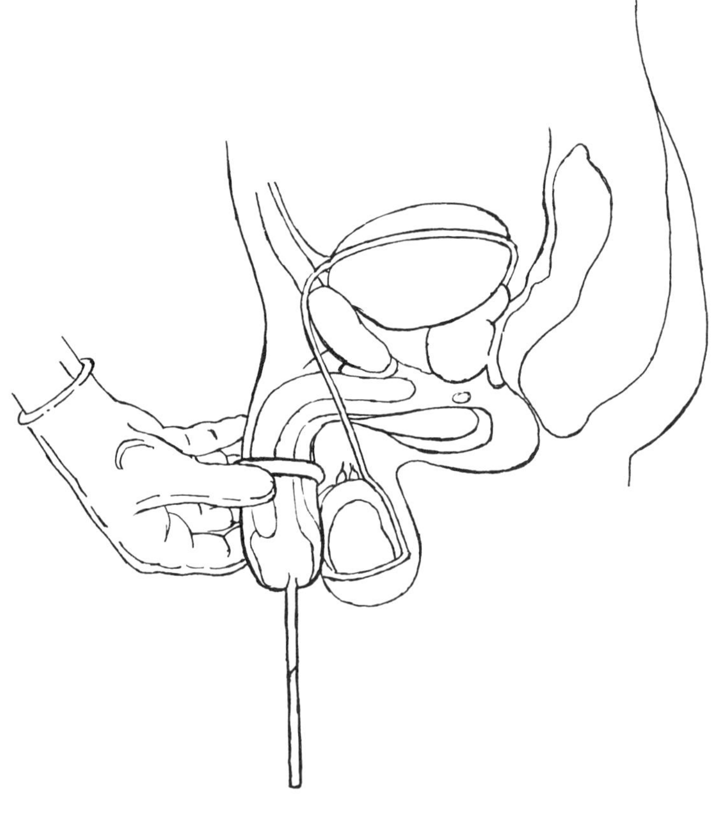

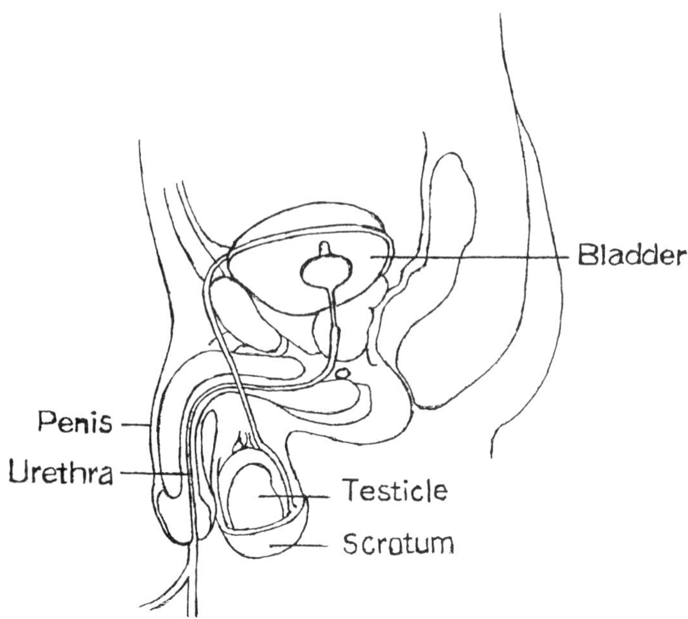

Male Catheterization

- The condom or Texas catheter is a specific type of catheter that can be used on male patients with a high susceptibility to urinary tract infections.
- The **condom catheter** has a condom-type device attached to the proximal end. The condom fits over and adheres to the penis.
- If urinary tract infections are not of concern, the Foley catheter is most commonly used.
- The male catheterization procedure is similar to that for the female. **Strict asepsis and sterile technique** should be employed.
- When cleansing with antiseptic solution, the imaging professional should **cleanse** from the meatus outward in circular motions.
- It may be necessary to cleanse and move foreskin back away from the meatus when performing this procedure on uncircumcised patients.
- The penis should be gripped firmly, and a generous amount of lubricant should be used when **inserting** the catheter.
- It is important to realize that the male urethra is approximately 14 to18 cm in length, considerably longer than the female urethra.
- The bladder is reached when urine begins to flow through the catheter. **Advance** the catheter at least 2 cm further and inflate the balloon with sterile water in order to secure the catheter.
- The catheter should be secured, with no tension on the tubing, to the groin area.

Removal of an Indwelling Catheter

- The most important consideration when removing a catheter is to **deflate the balloon.**
- Most catheters contain 10 ml of sterile water, but some require up to 30 ml.

- In order to properly drain the balloon, the size and type of catheter must be investigated.
- The patient's chart should be reviewed to observe any requests to record the amount of urine.
- If **measurement of output** is requested, it should be done after removing the catheter by draining all urine from the catheter and tubing into the bag and recording the total amount collected.
- The lumen, which acts to deflate the balloon, should never be cut, but a syringe should be attached and used to **withdraw the water.**
- The procedure requires the use of disposable gloves, paper towels, and a trash receptacle.
- The imaging professional should grasp the distal portion of the catheter as it is eased from the bladder.
- Wrap the catheter in a paper towel and dispose of the entire catheter apparatus in a contaminated-waste container.

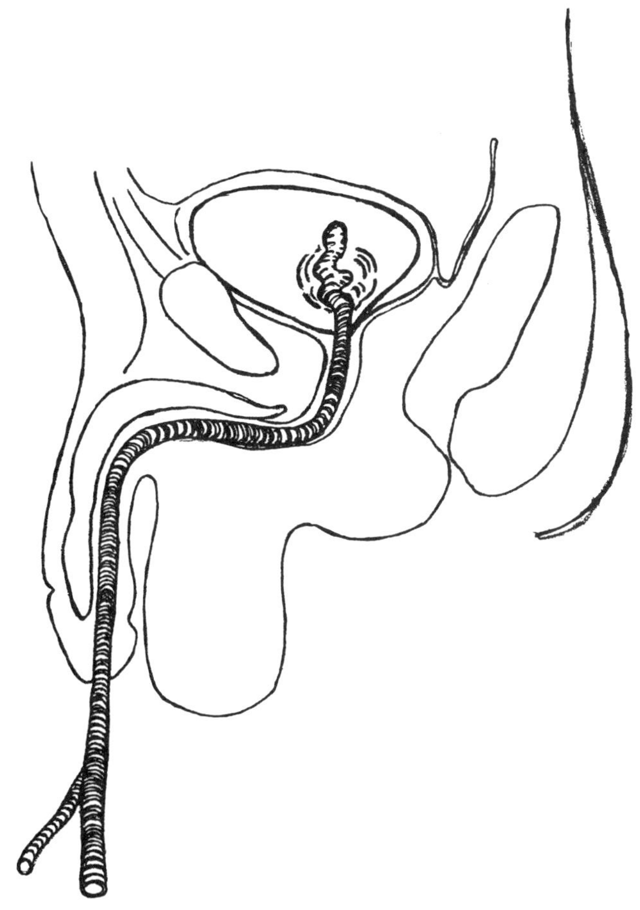

Considerations for the Imaging Professional

- Never drain a catheter bag, as urine output is usually measured.
- Keep the drainage bag below the level of the bladder at all times in order to prevent contamination duc to backflow.

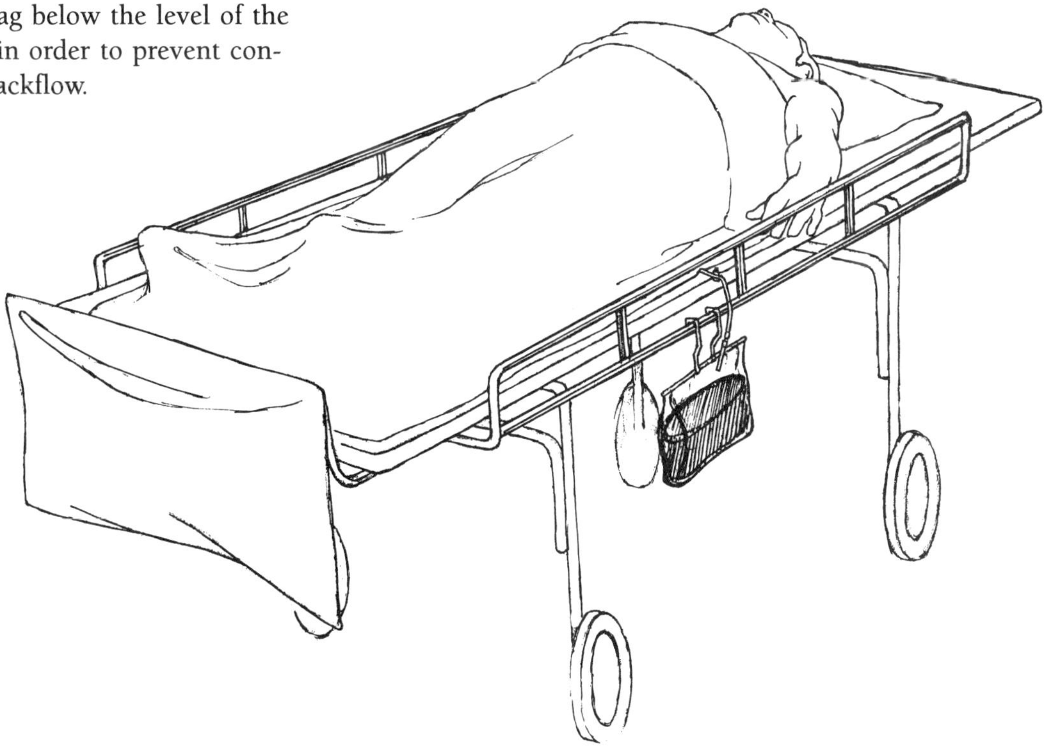

- Clamp tubing only if required by the specific imaging procedure or if the drainage bag must be raised above the level of the bladder.
- Drainage tubing should always be observed for kinks. for tension. and to ensure that it does not fall below the level of the drainage system.
- When transporting a patient with an indwelling catheter, the drainage system should be attached to the frame of the wheelchair or gurney at a point lower than the bladder.

Chapter 9 Review Questions

1. **Which type of gastric tube extends from the nose to the stomach and has a double lumen?**
   a. Levin
   b. gastric sump
   c. nasoenteric
   d. Dobhoff
2. **Which of type of tube is used to feed patients who cannot ingest orally?**
   a. gastric sump
   b. NG tube
   c. Dobhoff
   d. any of the above
3. **Which of the following is a surgically placed tube?**
   a. Dobhoff
   b. Levin
   c. Nutriflex
   d. jejunostomy
4. **When is a gastrostomy tube indicated?**
   a. when a patient cannot feed orally
   b. when there is a risk for reflux aspiration
   c. when a patient is immobile
   d. a and b only
   e. b and c only
   f. all of the above

5. **Which of the following methods should be used when gastric suction is necessary?**
   a. low continuous suction
   b. low sporadic suction
   c. high continuous suction
   d. low continuous suction

6. **Which of the following is not an indication for NG tube placement?**
   a. to prevent vomiting and reflux aspiration
   b. to secure a route for oral feeding
   c. to flush out ingested toxins
   d. to drain the stomach contents

7. **When separated, which of the following can cause a pneumothorax?**
   a. parietal pleura
   b. visceral pleura
   c. epidural pleura
   d. a and c only
   e. a and b only

8. **Air that collects and becomes trapped in the pleural space is specifically termed a**
   a. pneumothorax.
   b. hemothorax.
   c. closed pneumothorax.
   d. closed hemothorax.

9. **Chest tubes are inserted via**
   a. any open wound.
   b. an incision through the diaphragm.
   c. a thoracotomy into the chest.
   d. the trachea.

10. **Which of the following is the main purpose of the water seal drainage system?**
    a. to help secure the chest tube
    b. to allow air to escape the pleural cavity
    c. as a method of irrigation
    d. all of the above

11. **When transporting a patient with a water seal apparatus via a wheelchair, where should the device be placed?**
    a. in the patient's lap
    b. hooked onto the back of the wheelchair
    c. below the level of the chest
    d. The water seal system should be unhooked prior to transport.

12. **Which of the following is not a true statement?**
    a. Urinary catheterization requires strict asepsis.
    b. Urinary catheterization is a sterile procedure.
    c. Sterile gloves are not necessary.
    d. The urinary bladder is sterile.

13. **What evidence indicates that a catheter has reached the bladder?**
    a. The catheter cannot be advanced any further.
    b. The patient gives an indication.
    c. The catheter becomes easier to advance.
    d. Urine begins to flow back through the catheter.

14. **Which of the following should be used to inflate the balloon securing a catheter in the bladder?**
    a. oxygen
    b. air
    c. sterile water
    d. tap water

15. **When is a condom catheter necessary?**
    a. if a patient is pregnant
    b. if a male patient is susceptible to bladder infections
    c. if a Foley catheter is not readily available
    d. if there is trauma to the kidneys

16. **What is the most important step to remember when removing an indwelling catheter?**
    a. Deflate the balloon.
    b. Remove it using one constant movement.
    c. Wear sterile gloves.
    d. Do not allow urine to drip onto the floor.

Venipuncture and Routes of Drug Administration

CHAPTER 10

VENIPUNCTURE

- **Venipuncture** is the process of inserting a needle or catheter into a vein, usually to withdraw blood for analysis.
- The **process** of venipuncture can be achieved with the use of a syringe or a Vacutainer system.

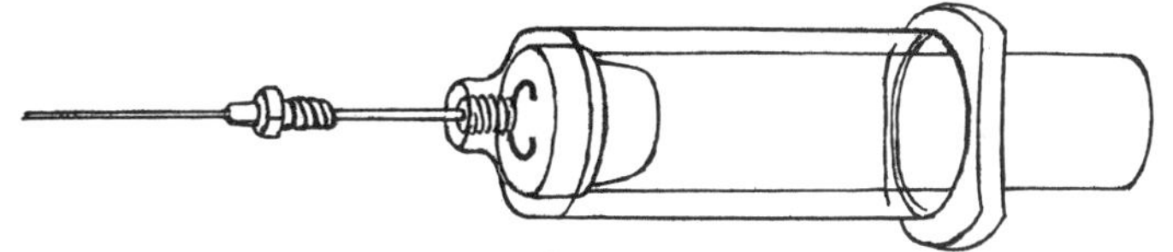

- A **syringe** is commonly used in the imaging department when injecting contrast for radiographic examinations.
- A **Vacutainer system** is most commonly used when various types of analysis will be performed requiring the collection of more than one sample.
- The system allows vacuum-sealed collection tubes, after being inserted into a plastic guide, to be punctured, permitting the collection of a blood specimen.
- The needle and plastic guide must be kept sterile.
- Disposable gloves and medical asepsis should be utilized.
- When **choosing the puncture site**, it is important to note the convenience and condition of the vein.
- **Common sites** for insertion of the needle include the basilic vein, median cubital vein, cephalic vein, and median antebrachial vein.
- Once the vein is located, a tourniquet should be tied around the patient's arm above the elbow. The tourniquet should be left on for a minimal amount of time.

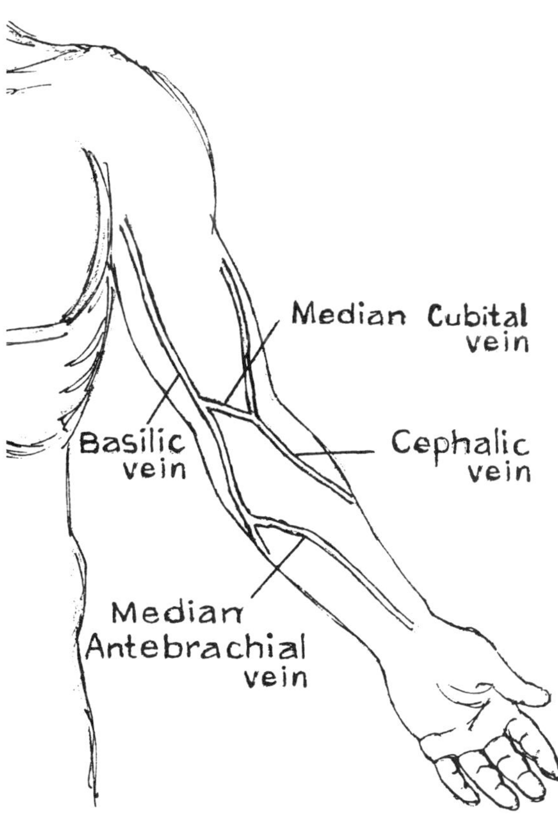

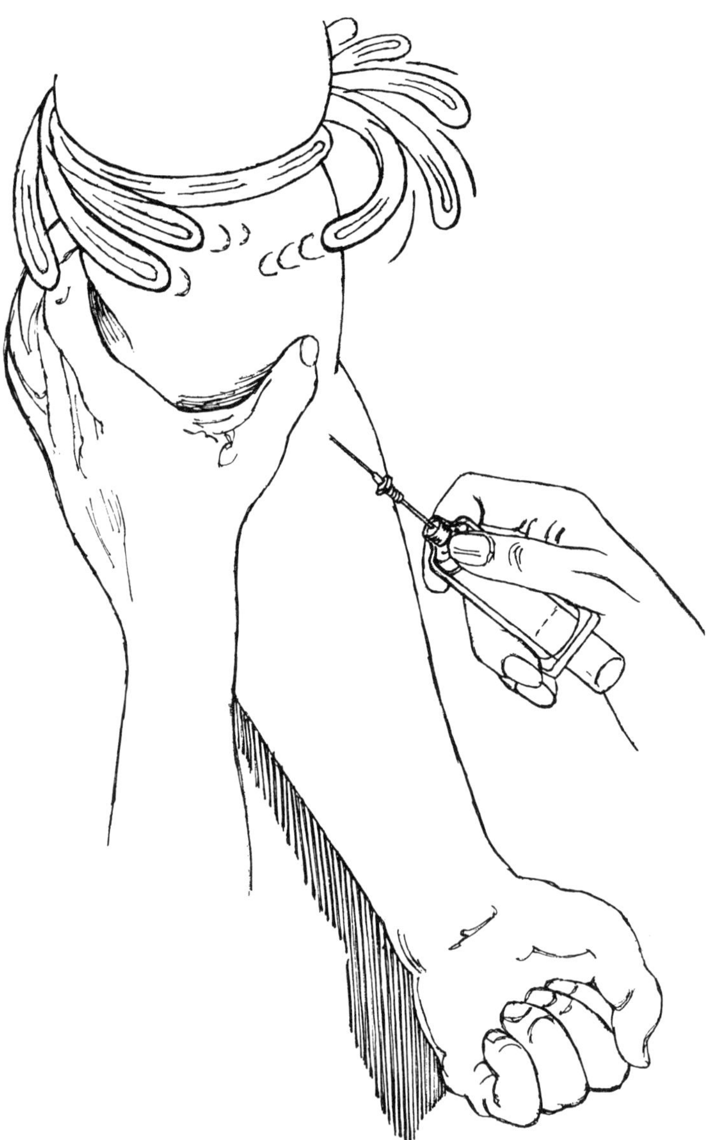

- The site should be cleansed with antiseptic and allowed to dry to avoid burning by the antiseptic at the puncture site.
- The needle should be **inserted** with the bevel up, parallel to the vein, at a 35-45-degree angle using a slow, constant motion. It is important that the needle not be advanced through the vein.
- The tourniquet should be removed once the needle is inserted into the vein.
- When removing the specimen tube, it is imperative that the plastic holder be grasped firmly in order to prevent accidental extraction of the needle.
- If using the **Vacutainer system**, once the needle is in the vein, the specimen container should be pushed onto the plastic container which will puncture the stopper and allow blood to flow into the container.
- If using a **syringe**, once blood is seen at the base of the stopper, the stopper can be pulled to draw blood into the syringe.
- A **small bandage** should be placed over the puncture site on removal of the needle with minimal compression being applied.
- All equipment should be disposed of in a sharps container.
- **Needles should not be bent, broken, or recapped before discarding.**

PARENTERAL INJECTION

- Medications administered parenterally are given through a subcutaneous, intramuscular, intradermal, or intravenous route.
- Other routes that physicians may use to administer medications are intra-arterial, intrathecal, and intra-articular.
- **Reasons** for parenteral administration of medications include the following:
  - An emergency situation requiring swift drug action
  - Inability of the patient to tolerate oral routes of medication
  - Need to localize anesthesia or focus the medication to a precise area of the body
  - Situations in which digestion could counter the effects of the medication.

Subcutaneous Routes

- **Subcutaneous** (SC) routes of administration are utilized to introduce medication to tissues below the dermal layer.
- Methods of injection usually involve a needle with a smaller lumen at a 45- to 90-degree angle depending on the site.
- Common **sites** of subcutaneous injection include the deltoid muscle and upper thigh, which contain extensive capillary beds that absorb medication quickly.

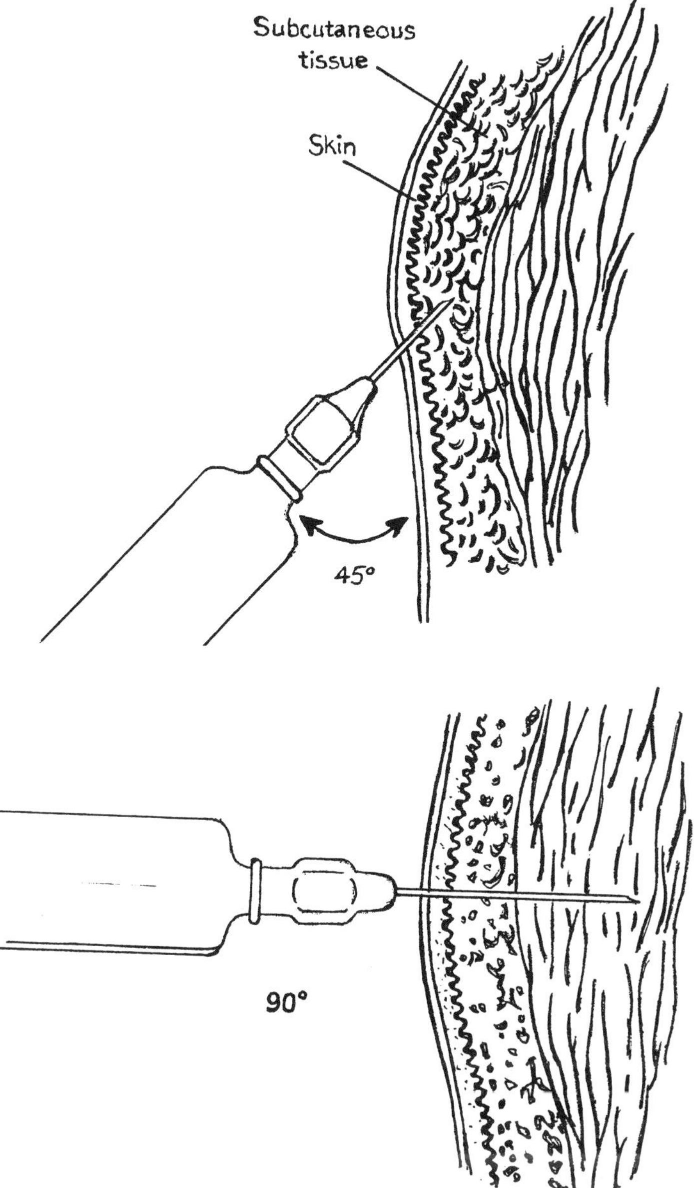

Intramuscular Administration

- **Intramuscular** (IM) injections deploy medication into the muscular layer which can tolerate larger amounts with less discomfort.
- Most commonly the method of administration is with a 22- to 23-gauge 1½- to 3-inch needle at a 90-degree angle.
- **Sites** for intramuscular injections include the deltoid, gluteal, and lateral and ventral muscles of the thigh.

Intradermal Route

- The **intradermal** route is commonly used for skin testing because small amounts of medication can be deposited under the skin.
- The mode of administration is with a needle with a small lumen, 25 gauge or less, and a 10-degree angle insertion.
- The most common **site** is on the volar surface of the arm.

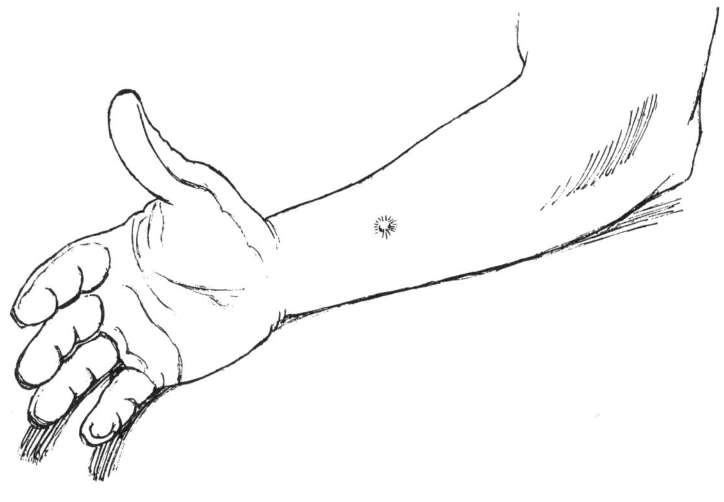

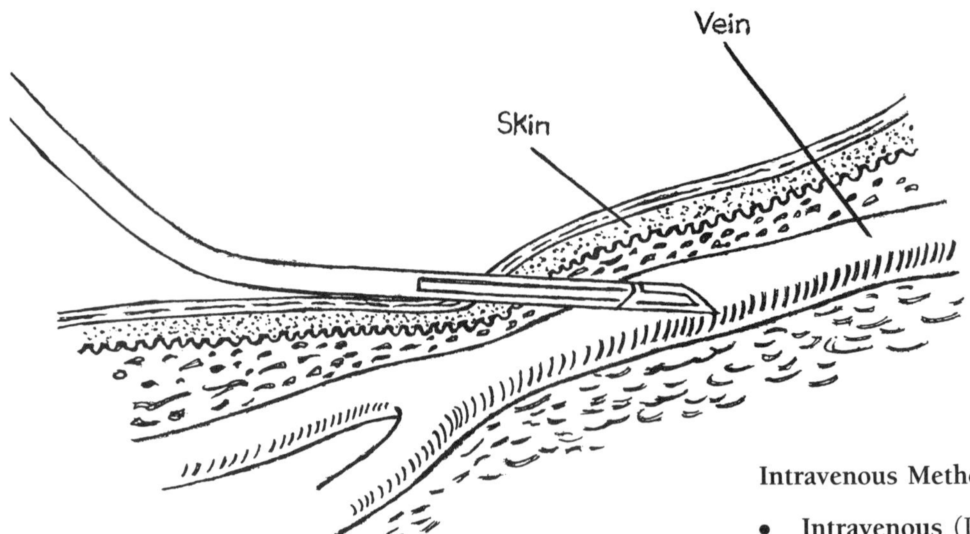

Intravenous Method

- **Intravenous** (IV) medications provide a direct route to the bloodstream for medication or fluid. This method is the swiftest of all routes.
- The mode of insertion is similar to that for venipuncture, using a needle between 18 and 22 gauge depending on the viscosity of the medication being injected.
- **Most commonly** the veins of the arms are preferred for intravenous injection or insertion of an intravenous line.
- All material supplied intravenously must be **sterile** because it travels directly through the bloodstream.
- Because the route is directly through the bloodstream, it is advantageous in emergency situations.
- If an intravenous route must be used for an extended period, **butterfly needles** and more flexible plastic cannulas are preferred.

Other Routes of Administration

- **Topical routes** of drug administration include the skin, mucosa of the lungs, eyes, ears, nasopharynx, throat, rectum, and vagina.
- **Inhalants** for respiratory distress, eyedrops, suppositories, and topical antibiotics for skin ailments are examples of topical medications.
- **Enteral** or **oral** routes may be oral, sublingual, or rectal.
- The **oral** (PO) route is the easiest for most patients yet requires that the drug not be affected by gastric juices and not require direct action.

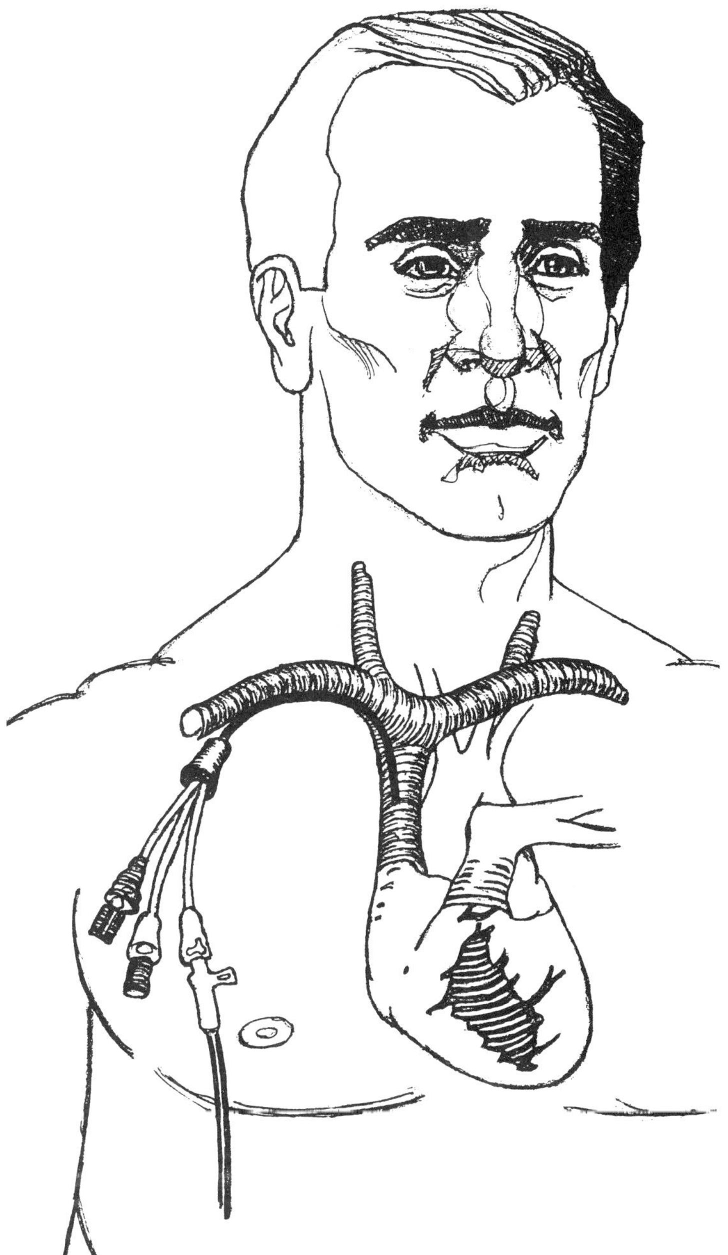

- Drugs administered **sublingually** are placed under the tongue and are absorbed into the bloodstream instantly, without gastric interaction.
- Oral nitroglycerin is an example of medication administered by the sublingual route.
- **Rectal** drug administration is used when patients cannot tolerate oral techniques, are vomiting, or are too young to swallow medications.
- Suppositories and enemas are examples of rectal drug administration.
- **Central venous catheters** and implanted **infusion ports** are common methods of IV therapy because they infuse solutions directly into the vascular system and are more difficult to dislodge.
- **Infusion ports** are primarily used for long-term drug therapy and require subcutaneous surgical implantation into the chest or intraspinal or intraperitoneal area.
- **Central venous methods**, or central lines, include the Swan-Ganz, Hickman, peripheral inserted (PIC), and Groshong catheters.
- **Purposes** of using a central venous catheter include intravenous nourishment, drug therapy, and chemotherapy.
- Long-term central venous catheter placement is usually into the **superior vena cava** by way of surgical implantation.
- Short-term central venous catheter placement is usually into the **jugular or subclavian vein.**

Considerations for the Imaging Professional

- Written orders must be confirmed before any drugs or medications are administered.
- Honest and informative communication with the patient should be practiced.
- Sterile, disposable needles should be utilized when administering injections.

- Needles should never be recapped, bent, broken, or removed from the syringe. They should always be disposed of in a specific sharps container.
- The administration of all drugs requires medical asepsis and surgical technique to prevent infection.
- When selecting an injection site, study the anatomy carefully to avoid causing blemishes, lesions, dermatitis, or other irritations.
- Shave the area if required to avert possible infection due to lodging of hair in the underlying tissue.
- Medications are absorbed at a higher rate through incisions or open tissue than when oral methods are used.
- Assistance may be required or an immobilizing device manufactured precisely for parenteral administration may be necessary.
- The proper rate of infusion should be maintained for IV therapy. The normal rate of infusion is 1 drop every 3 seconds.
- Infusion into a central venous or infusion port should be performed under the direct supervision of a physician and may require particular types of needles and solutions.
- Modification of technical factors may be necessary to visualize central venous lines radiographically when verifying correct placement.

Chapter 10 Review Questions

1. **When withdrawing blood for analysis, which of the following is most commonly used?**
   a. Vacutainer system
   b. butterfly needle
   c. direct stick
   d. syringe

2. **When choosing a puncture site, which of the following should be of primary concern?**

   I. **condition of the vein**
   II. **convenience of the site**
   III. **size of the vein**

   a. only I
   b. I and II only
   c. II and III only
   d. I and III only

3. **Which of the following is not a common site used for venipuncture?**
   a. cephalic vein
   b. median cubital vein
   c. femoral vein
   d. median antebrachial vein

4. **Which of the following is an incorrect statement about insertion of a needle for venipuncture?**
   a. The bevel should be up.
   b. The needle should be parallel to the vein.
   c. Insertion should be at a 45-degree angle.
   d. The tourniquet should be removed after the needle is removed from the vein.

5. **Which of the following is not a parenteral route for medication administration?**
   a. intramuscular
   b. rectal
   c. intradermal
   d. intravenous

6. **When administering subcutaneous medications, which of the following lumen sizes is not used?**
   a. 18 gauge
   b. 21 gauge
   c. 23 gauge
   d. 25 gauge

7. **Which of the following is a common reason for injecting medications into a muscle?**
   a. IM routes help alleviate nausea.
   b. IM routes are the quickest way to inject medication.
   c. IM routes allow larger amounts of medication to be employed with less discomfort.
   d. IM routes are the easiest for the health care provider to locate.

8. **Which of the following is a common reason for intradermal injection?**
   a. annual PPD testing
   b. polio vaccination
   c. mumps measles and rubella vaccination
   d. hepatitis B vaccination

9. The swiftest route for introducing medication into the bloodstream is which of the following?

a. intramuscular
b. intravenous
c. subcutaneous
d. intradermal

10. Which of the following is not an enteral route of medication?

a. oral
b. sublingual
c. rectal
d. topical

11. Which of the following is a common reason for administering medications rectally?

a. The patient cannot tolerate oral ingestion.
b. The patient is too young to ingest medication.
c. The patient is vomiting.
d. All of the above.
e. Only a and b.

12. Which of the following is used for long-term placement of a central venous catheter?

a. superior vena cava
b. jugular vein
c. subclavian vein
d. all of the above

Pharmacology, Drug Administration, and Radiographic Agents

CHAPTER 11

PHARMACOLOGY

- **Pharmacology** is a branch of science that studies drugs, their uses, their composition, and their interaction.
- The **divisions** of pharmacology include
  Pharmacokinetics
  Pharmacodynamics
  Pharmacognosy
  Toxicology
  Pharmacotherapeutics.
- Most relevant to radiographers are pharmacokinetics and pharmacodynamics.
- **Pharmacokinetics** investigates the metabolic, distribution, and absorption processes of the drug within the body.
- The **absorption** of a drug depends on the type of drug and how it is administered.
- Age, genetic composition, and disease processes may affect the rate at which the body metabolizes a drug.
- **Distribution** of a drug pertains to how it is dispersed thoughout the body. Organs with a high rate of blood flow receive more exposure to the drug.
- **Pharmacodynamics** deals with specific effects or actions of a particular drug.
- **Effects** of a drug are influenced by such factors as the patient's weight, gender, age, emotions, current physical state, and genetic make-up.
- Most drugs are taken at specified times in order to maintain continuous action of the medication.

- Severe reactions to a drug are usually termed adverse reactions and are classified as allergic, idiosyncratic, and iatrogenic.
- **Allergic reactions** are caused by an antigen-antibody reaction and may exhibit mild symptoms such as a rash or severe symptoms such as vasoconstriction and death.
- **Idiosyncratic reactions** are categorized as unusual responses that are not allergic in nature and may be due to genetic or hormonal influences.
- Drug-induced diseases or manifestations are classified as **iatrogenic responses**.

DRUG CLASSIFICATION

- Drugs can be classified by their **clinical effect on the body** or by their **effect on a specific system**.
- The choice of drugs used is dependent on the specific symptoms or disease manifestations.
- **Antibiotics** are used to eradicate infection caused by bacteria, parasites, or fungi.
- **Complications** of antibiotics may include
  Secondary infection
  Developed resistance
  Tissue damage or injury
  Hypersensitivity or an allergic reaction.
- **Central nervous system** (CNS) medications fall into two categories: stimulants and depressants.
- Sedatives, narcotics, antianxiety drugs, antidepressants, and antipsychotics are some of the types of drugs used to treat the CNS.
- Medications used in **peripheral nervous system** treatment consist of anticoagulants, hemostatics, vasodilators, analgesics, and antiarrhythmics.
- Nasal decongestants, antihistamines, and antitussives are drugs that are used in conjunction with **respiratory system disorders**.
- **Gastrointestinal system** medications include antacids, stool softeners, antidiarrheals, laxatives, anticholinergics, and antiemetics.
- Anticoagulants, antihypertensives, diuretics, hemostatics, and antianginals are heart and **circulatory system** medications.

- The accompanying chart lists drugs by body system, action, and name. It is not a complete listing and is not based on preference.

Chosen Drugs Compiled by Body System, Action, and Name

System Classification	Drug Action	Drug Name
Antiinfectious		
Antibiotics	Discourage or kill microorganisms	Erythromycin, cephalosporin, penicillin, tetracycline
Antiseptics	Discourage growth of microbes on tissue	Hydrogen peroxide, isopropyl alcohol, povidone iodine
Central nervous system		
Sedatives	Relieve anxiety, promote sleep	Chloral hydrate, phenobarbital, secobarbital, triazolam
Narcotics	Alleviate modest to oppressive pain	Codeine, hydromorphone, meperidine, morphine
Antianxiety	Ease anxiety	Alprazolam, Buspirone, Lorazepam, Chlordiazepoxide
Antidepressants	Help relieve depression	Amitriptyline, doxepin, fluoxteine, sertraline
Antipsychotics	Lessen and relieve psychotic symptoms	Chlorpromazine, clozapine, haloperidol
Peripheral nervous system		
Anti-inflammatory analgesics	Reduce mild to moderate pain and inflammation	Ibuprofen, naproxen, piroxicam
Other analgesics	Reduce mild to moderate pain and fever	Acetaminophen, aspirin, propoxyphene
Antiarrhythmics	Manage the heart rate	Atropine, lidocaine, quinidine
Anticoagulants	Discourage blood clotting	Heparine, sodium warfarin
Hemostatics	Encourage blood clotting	Gel foam, vitamin K
Vasodilators	Increase blood flow peripherally	Hydralazine, minoxidil
Respiratory system		
Antihistamines	Reduce congestion and inhibit allergic reactions	Diphenhydramine hydrochloride, dimenhydrinate
Antitussives	Reduce and relieve cough	Codeine, dextromethorphan, guaifenesin
Bronchodilators	Ease breathing in asthma and severe allergic reactions	Epinephrine (Adrenalin), Ephedrine, Albuterol
Nasal decongestants	Ease rhinitis due to sinus infections, allergies, and colds	Phenylpropanolamine, Pseudoephedrine
Gastrointestinal system		
Antacids	Neutralize stomach acids	Aluminum and magnesium hydroxides, sodium bicarbonate
Antidiarrheals	Reduce bowel movements and agitation	Diphenoxylate, kaolin, pectin
Antiemetics	Alleviate nausea and repress vomiting	Benzquinamide, prochlorperazine
Anticholinergics	Reduce stomach secretions and spasms	Atropine, propantheline mepenzolate
Laxatives	Soften and promote bowel movements	Magnesium citrate, castor oil, milk of magnesia
Circulatory system		
Antianginals	Increase blood flow to the heart	Nifedipine, nitroglycerin
Antihypertensives	Manage high blood pressure	Atenolol, captopril, clonidine
Diuretics	Reduce edema	Furosemide, Mannitol, Thiazides

RADIOGRAPHIC CONTRAST AGENTS

- Radiographic contrast agents are frequently used when imaging specific organs or body systems.
- There are two basic types of contrast agents, positive and negative.
- **Positive contrast agents** can be administered orally, vaginally, rectally, intravenously, intra-arterially, or intrathecally.
- Because of their high atomic number, positive contrast agents interrupt photons as they travel toward the film.
- Thus, positive contrast agents provide light areas or areas of "contrast" on the radiographic image.
- Common **types** of positive contrast include iodinated contrast and barium sulfate.
- **Negative contrast agents** do not interrupt photon travel and have very low atomic numbers.
- **Air** is the most common negative contrast agent used in radiography. Carbon dioxide, oxygen, and nitrous oxide are also negative contrast agents.
- Common **uses** of negative contrast include air employed in barium enema studies and in arthrography.
- Contrast agents are considered drugs because they may elicit a physiological response when administered.
- The most common contrast agents are air, iodinated products and barium sulfate.

Iodinated Contrast Media

- An **iodinated contrast** medium is commonly used in studies involving the urinary, circulatory, and central nervous systems.
- As iodine composition increases, atomic number and the ability to opacify structures increases.
- The **two types** of iodinated contrast media are water-soluble and oil-based.

- A **water-soluble contrast** medium is used most frequently, as it is the only type of contrast agent that can be injected into the bloodstream.
- Water-soluble contrast agents are excreted from the body via the urinary system.
- Common **forms** of water-soluble contrast agents are ionic and nonionic media.
- **Nonionic** agents produce less reaction and are less toxic because of their lower osmotic capability.
- **Osmolarity** is a term that describes the number of particles in a specific type of solution.
- **Ionic** contrast media have greater potential for adverse effects because of their higher osmolarity.
- Contrast media can penetrate blood cells. Those with higher osmolarity penetrate blood cells at a higher rate than those with low osmolarity.
- **Penetration of blood cells** can cause a displacement of body fluids that may be responsible for adverse patient reactions.
- **Reactions** to contrast media experienced by the patient are, in order of severity, as follows:
  Nausea, headache, metallic taste in the mouth
  Hives, itchy throat and nose
  Cough, vomiting, wheezing, chest pain
  Death.
- Most reactions to contrast media occur within **5 minutes** of administration. It is essential that the imaging professional stay with the patient during procedures involving contrast agents.
- In order to reduce the possibility of a reaction to a contrast agent, a thorough **patient history** should be obtained. The following information should be included:
  Allergy history, including medications, foods, asthma, and hay fever
  Prior contrast history
  Current list of medications the patient is taking
  Vital signs and lab results.
- **Oil-based contrast agents** can be used for specific studies of the female reproductive system and the lymph systems.

SUNNYSIDE COMMUNITY HOSPITAL
DIAGNOSTIC IMAGING DEPARTMENT

Referred by Dr. ____________________

PLEASE ANSWER THE FOLLOWING:

1. Are you allergic to any medication?
No ______ Yes ______ Please list ______________________________

2. Are you allergic to any local anesthetics?
No ______ Yes ______ Please list if known ______________________________

3. Do you have any other known allergies?
(asthma, severe hay fever, food allergies, etc.)
____
____

4. Is there any specific allergy to iodine or seafood? ______________________________
____

5. Have you ever had an angiogram (arteriogram), kidney x-ray test (IVP), gallbladder x-ray or CT Scan before?
No ______ Yes ______ If so, any adverse side effects or reactions? ______________________________
Specify ______________________________

6. Are you currently taking glucophage (Metformin) or any other medication for diabetes?
No ______ Yes ______ Please list if known ______________________________

PLEASE DO NOT WRITE BELOW THIS LINE UNTIL OUR RADIOLOGIST VISITS WITH YOU

I. I give Dr. ______________________________ permission to perform the following test on me:
____

II. I certify that Dr. ______________________________ has discussed with me the above listed procedure and that I understand the hoped for benefits. I further certify that I understand and accept the possible risks of said procedure, that I have read and understand the information in this form and consent to the performance of this procedure upon my person. I acknowledge that no warranty or guarantee can be made to me concerning results or cure.

Name ______________________________

Signature ______________________________

Relationship ______________________________

Date ______________________________ Time ______________________________ A.M. P.M.

Witness ______________________________

- This type of contrast cannot be injected into the bloodstream as it would cause embolism and death.
- Oil-based contrast agents are not commonly used at imaging facilities.

Considerations for the Imaging Professional

- Medications should never be given without the consent of the patient and on written orders of a physician.
- An analysis of current medications that may contraindicate contrast agents should be obtained before administering any drugs.
- Physical histories, including genetic anomalies, sensitivities to drugs, and allergies, should be documented.
- Patients receiving contrast media should be well hydrated to prevent toxicity.
- Patients should be instructed regarding possible symptoms of delayed reactions to contrast agents.
- Patients receiving contrast media should never be left unattended.
- Rapid administration of some contrast agents may lead to overdose and toxicity, causing severe damage to the liver and kidneys.
- Contrast agents should be protected from light and administered at body temperature using strict aseptic techniques.

IMAGING WITH RADIOGRAPHIC CONTRAST MEDIA

- **Barium sulfate ($BaSO_4$)** is the most common contrast medium used in studies involving the GI system.
- Because barium is a metal and is not water-soluble, it is not naturally absorbed by the body.

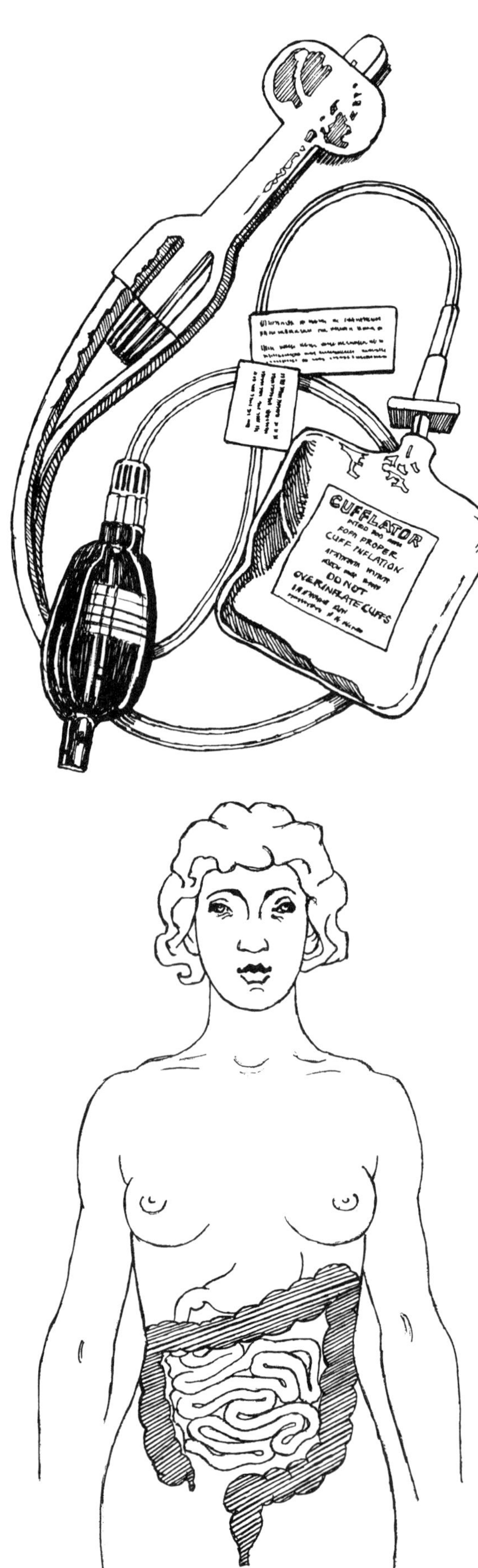

- $BaSO_4$ should never be injected into the circulatory system or subarachnoid space or used when perforation of the peritoneum is possible.
- **Barium enema studies** require the use of $BaSO_4$ and may also call for a negative contrast agent such as air or carbon dioxide.
- Visualization is usually of the large bowel from the rectum to the ileocecal region.
- It may be necessary to administer the drug **glucagon** in order to reduce gastric motility and prevent cramping.
- Most **equipment** used for this study comes prepackaged and includes a barium enema bag, enema tip (with an inflatable cuff), and an inflation pump.
- Water should be added to the enema bag of barium, followed by vigorous shaking to force the barium and water into suspension form.
- The suspension should be uniform in order to coat the bowel consistently.
- The bag is then hung, and barium is allowed to flow to the end of the tubing attached to the enema bag.
- To **insert** the enema tip the patient should be placed in Sims' position and an attempt should be made to ensure modesty.
- The enema tip located at the distal end of the tubing is inserted into the patient's rectum past the rectal sphincter. Note that allergies to latex may warrant the use of a special type of enema tip.
- Once past the rectal sphincter, the **cuff or balloon** is carefully inflated to secure the tip within the rectum. No amount of force should be necessary to insert the enema tip.
- The radiologist then fills the bowel with barium and possibly air to visualize the lower GI tract.
- Fluoroscopic films, spot films, and plain radiographs may be taken to evaluate the system.
- Before removing the rectal tip, the imaging professional should allow the barium to drain into the enema bag by placing it below the level of the rectum.

- The rectal tip should then be removed by **deflating the cuff** and gently easing it from the rectum.
- If evaluation must be performed on a patient with a **surgical stoma**, the patient should be instructed to bring an extra ostomy pouch.
- Inserting the enema tip and performing barium studies on patients with intestinal stomas requires evaluation of the specific location and type of colostomy or ileostomy.
- **Strict aseptic technique** should be employed to prevent infection of the surgical site.

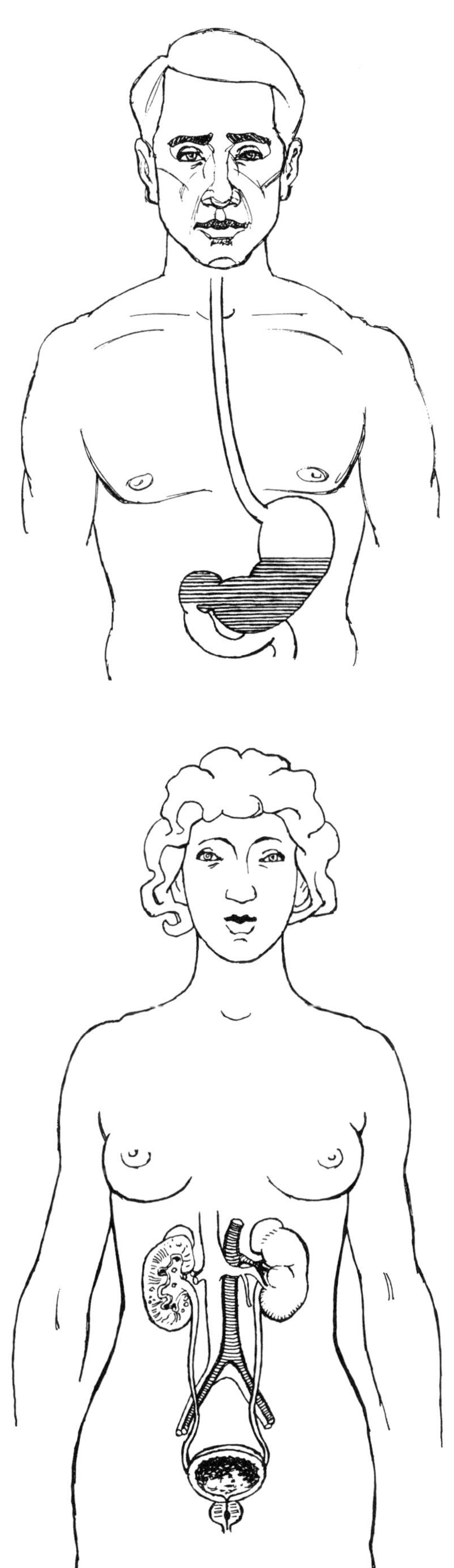

Upper Gastrointestinal Studies

- An **upper gastrointestinal** (**UGI**) study is used to evaluate the pharynx, esophagus, stomach, and small bowel.
- Glucagon may be indicated for this study. Possible adverse reactions to glucagon include nausea, vomiting, and hives.
- Oral ingestion of flavored $BaSO_4$ is used for this procedure. Sodium bicarbonate, in crystal form, may also be required for **double-contrast studies.**
- The barium is swallowed and allowed to pass through the GI tract.
- Fluoroscopic films, spot films, and plain radiographs may be taken to evaluate the system.
- If a **small bowel examination** is also requested, additional film will be required at fixed intervals as indicated by the radiologist.
- It may be necessary to perform a UGI examination on patients with an NG tube.
- If the patient cannot drink the $BaSO_4$, it can be administered using a syringe which allows evaluation of the stomach and small bowel.

Urinary System Imaging

- An **intravenous pyelogram** (**IVP**) is the most common study of the urinary system requiring a contrast agent.
- Iodinated contrast is used for this procedure and is injected intravenously.

- A complete history, including past contrast studies, a physical history, drugs taken, and current and past illnesses should be obtained.
- The patient must **sign a consent** form allowing the injection of radiographic contrast for the procedure.
- An IVP provides information to aid in the diagnosis of conditions involving the kidneys, ureters, bladder, and urethra.
- **Other examinations** performed on the urinary system requiring iodinated contrast may include the cystogram and variations thereof, the nephrogram, and the urethrogram.
- Once the contrast medium is injected, it travels through the venous system and is filtered through the kidneys.
- Radiographs are taken of the urinary system at specified intervals which highlight the structures of interest.
- When performing an IVP on patients with an indwelling urinary catheter, the **catheter should be clamped** in order to achieve filling of the bladder.
- Patients receiving iodinated contrast should be carefully monitored for symptoms of anaphylaxis.
- Dehydration, impaired renal function, and an allergy to iodinated contrast are **contraindications** for the IVP examination.

Required Preparations for Contrast Procedures

Barium Enema

- A barium enema involves a **24-hour preparation** which may include laxatives and cleansing enemas to remove all fecal material from the bowel.
- The patient should have a liquid dinner the night prior to the examination.
- Nothing should be taken by mouth (NPO) after midnight prior to the examination.
- The patient should be instructed not to smoke, chew gum, or brush his teeth, as this stimulates GI secretions.

- If the patient has conditions that require medication, the radiologist should be consulted to evaluate scheduling as well as ingestion of medication prior to the study.

Upper Gastrointestinal and Urinary System Studies

- The UGI and IVP examinations usually require a **12-hour preparation.**
- The patient should be instructed to have a light meal the night prior to the examination.
- A cleansing enema may be necessary for patients having an IVP examination.
- Nothing should be taken by mouth (NPO) after midnight prior to the examination.
- The patient should be instructed not to smoke, chew gum or brush her teeth, as this stimulates GI secretions.
- If the patient has conditions requiring medication, the radiologist should be consulted to evaluate scheduling as well as ingestion of medication prior to the study.

Considerations for the Imaging Professional

- Examinations using contrast should be performed as follows:
  1. All noncontrast studies should be carried out prior to examinations involving contrast.
  2. Studies using iodinated contrast should be completed prior to barium studies.
  3. Barium studies of the lower GI tract should be completed before those involving the upper GI tract.
  4. Scheduling of examinations that require the patient to take nothing by mouth should be completed early in the morning.
  5. When scheduling procedures, special consideration should be given to pediatric patients, elderly patients, and patients who have diabetes or are on explicit drug therapy
- Patients should be instructed to drink plenty of water following barium studies of the GI tract in order to prevent obstruction.
- Proper instructions for preparation for the examination should be given, in writing if possible, to patients.

SUNNYSIDE COMMUNITY HOSPITAL
10TH & TACOMA • P.O. BOX 719
SUNNYSIDE, WASHINGTON 98944

STEWART COLE, D.O., RADIOLOGIST VIVIENNE KEZUKA, D.O., RADIOLOGIST

DIAGNOSTIC IMAGING DEPARTMENT

X-RAY — ULTRASOUND — MAMMOGRAPHY

(509) 837-1760

NAME: ______________________ REFERRING PHYSICIAN: ______________________

APPT. DATE: ______________________ BUN*: ______________________

APPT. TIME: ______________________ CREATINE*: ______________________

PATIENT HISTORY: ____

____

EXAMINATION REQUESTED: LMP: ______________________

X-RAY			FINGER		RIBS BILAT.		UGI		PREGNANCY COMPLETE
	ABDOMEN (KUB)		FOOT		RIBS UNILAT.		UGI & SB		PREGNANCY F/U
	ABDOMEN 2VWS		FOREARM		S-I JOINTS		VOIDING CYSTOGRAM		SONO. AORTA
	ABDOMEN 3VWS		G.B. ORAL		SACRUM & COCCYX		WRIST		SONO. GALLBLADDER
	A-C JOINT		HAND		SCAPULA		ZYGOMATIC ARCH		SONO. KIDNEY UNIL.
	ANKLE		HIP BILAT.		SCOLIOSIS STUDY	**ULTRASOUND**			SONO. LIVER
	BARIUM ENEMA		HIP UNILAT.		SHOULDER		ABDOMEN COMPLETE		SONO. PANCREAS
	B.E. W/AIR		HIPS INFANT		SINUSES WATERS VW		AORTA/IVC		SONO. PROSTATE
	BONE AGE STUDY		HUMERUS		SINUSE SERIES		ART. UPPER EXT.		SONO. RETRO. COMPLETE
	BONE LENGTH		IVP HYPERTENSIVE		SKULL COMPLETE		ART. LOWER EXT.		SONO. SPLEEN
	C SPINE 2VWS		IVP W/TOMOS.		SKULL LIMITED		CAROTID BILAT.		SONO. TESTES
	C SPINE 5 VWS		KNEE 2VWS		SMALL BOWEL		CAROTID UNILAT.		SONO. THYROID
	C SPINE 7VWS		KNEE 3 VWS		S/T NECK 1VW		CAROTID F/U		U/S BREAST
	CHEST 1VW		L SPINE 3VWS		S/T NECK 2VWS		ECHO / TRANSVAGINAL		U/S EXT. NON-VASCULAR
	CHEST 2VWS		L SPINE 5VWS		STANDING POSTURAL		FETAL AGE REPEAT		U/S GUIDED NDLE BIO.
	CHEST LORDOTIC		L SPINE 7VWS		STERNUM		FETAL BIO-PROFILE		VENOUS DUPLEX BILAT.
	CLAVICLE		MANDIBLE		SWALLOW FUNCTION		INTRAUT. DEV. LOC.		VENOUS DUPLEX UNI.
	CYSTOGRAPHY		MASTOIDS		THORACOLUMBAR SPINE		OB COMPLT. MULT. GEST.	**MAMMOGRAPHY**	
	ELBOW		MET. BONE SURVEY		TIBIA/FIBULA		OB 1ST TRI.		MAMM SCREEN
	ESOPHAGUS		NASAL BONES		T-M JOINTS		OB LIMITED		MAMM BILAT. DIAG.
	EYE FOREIGN BODY		ORBITS		T SPINE 2VWS		PELVIC NON-OB		MAMM UNILAT. DIAG.
	FACIAL BONES		OS CALSIS		T SPINE 3 VWS		PELVIC F/U		MAMM UNILAT. F/U
	FEMUR		PELVIS		TOE		PLEURAL EFFUSION LOC.		NEEDLE LOC.

Reports are routinely placed in mail boxes or mailed.
If special handling is desired, check below.

☐ Return patient and films to my office now.

☐ "Wet Read" call Phone # ______________

REFER TO REVERSE FOR SPECIFIC INSTRUCTIONS
Referir al reves para instrucciónes específicos

SCH FORM NO. X-04C (REV. 1/96)

ADDRESSOGRAPH

PREPARATIONS & INSTRUCTIONS

☐ **UPPER GI SERIES (UGI) AND/OR SMALL BOWEL**

1. Take nothing by mouth from 12:00 p.m. on the night before the examination until you report here the following morning. This includes foods, liquids and medications. No smoking.
   No tome Vd. nada por la boca a partir de las 12:00 p.m. (medianoche) la noche antes del exámen hasta que Vd. venga al hospital el día siguiente; esto incluye los alimeñtos, líquidos y medicinas.

☐ **BARIUM ENEMA (BE)**

1. Nothing to eat or drink except fruit juices, starting 12:00 noon the day before the examination.
   No coma ni tome Vd. nada con la excepción de jugos de fruta. (a partir de las 12:00 [Mediodia] el día antes del examen)
2. 3 ounces of castor oil at 2:00 p.m. 2 Dulcolax at 7:00 p.m.
   Tome vd. 3 onzas de aceite de recino a las 2:00 p.m. 2 Dulcolax a las 7:00 p.m. de la tarde el día antes del exámen.
3. Nothing for breakfast except fruit juice.
   No coma Vd. nada en la mañana con la excepción de jugo de fruta.

☐ **ORAL GALLBLADDER (GB)**

1. Eat a light supper of dry toast, jelly and fruit juice.
   Como Vd. una cena ligera de pan tostado (seco), mermelada y jugo de fruta.
2. After the meal, begin taking the tablets, one every five minutes with enough water to wash them down.
   Después de la cena empieze Vd. a tomar las pastillas, una cada cinco minutos con el agua necesaria para pasarla.
3. From then on take nothing by mouth until the examination is completed the following morning.
   De ahora en adelante no tome Vd. nada por la boca hasta que Vd. termine con el exámen la mañana siguiente.

☐ **EXCRETORY UROGRAM — INTRAVENOUS PYELOGRAM (IVP)**

1. Nothing to eat or drink except fruit juices, starting 12:00 noon the day before the examination.
   No coma ni tome Vd. nada con la excepción de jugos de fruta.
2. 2 ounces Castor Oil 2 p.m. 2 Dulcolax 7:00 p.m.
   2 onzas de aciete de recino a las 2 de la tarde. 2 tabletas de Dulcolax a las 7:00 de la noche.
3. Nothing for breakfast except fruit juice.
   No coma Vd. nada en la mañana con la excepción de jugo de fruta.

☐ **MAMMOGRAPHY/MAMOGRAFIA**

1. On the day of the examination, do not use deodorant, perfume, powders, ointments or preparation of any sort on the breast area, or underarms. Residual on the skin from such preparations can obscure your films. Basic (routine, screening) mammograms take 30 minutes. All other mammography exams take 45 minutes.
   En el día de su examen, no use desodorante, perfumes, talco, cremas o morguna preparación en la area o en los pechos. Residuo en la piel de tal preparaciones pueden obscurecer en sus radiografías. Mamografias routinas duran media hora (30 minutos). Toda las otras mamografías pueden durar cuarenta y cinco minutos para tomarlas.

☐ **ULTRASOUND/ULTRASONIDO**

1. LIVER, GALLBLADDER, PANCREAS AND AORTA SCANS: Prep with Mylicon 80, 16 tablets. Take two with each meal and two at bedtime, starting 2 days before the exam. You should have nothing to eat or drink starting 12 hours before the exam.
   HIGADO, VESICULA, PANCREAS AND AORTA SCANS: Preparese con Mylicon 80, 16 tabletas. Tome dos con cada comida, y dos antes de acostarse, empesando dos días antes de su examen. No coma o beba doce (12) horas antes de su examen.
2. KIDNEY SCAN: Drink 16-24 ounces of fluid one hour prior to the exam. You may void.
   EXAMEN DE LOS RIÑONES: Tome diez y sies a viente-cuatro onzas de líquidos una hora antes de su examen. Orinar es permitido.
3. PELVIS AND OB/GYN SCANS: Drink 16-24 ounces of fluid at least one hour before the exam. DO NOT VOID. Your bladder must be very full at the time of the exam.
   Tome 16-24 onzas de líquido una hora antes de su examen. No orine. Necesita estar llena su vejiga al tiempo de su examen.

- Water-soluble contrast should be used for patients with possible bowel perforation or obstruction but may be contraindicated for those with an iodine allergy.
- Thorough explanation of the procedure should be provided to the patient with a careful explanation regarding the equipment and possible discomfort.

Chapter 11 Review Questions

1. **The study of the specific effects of a given medication is known as**
   a. pharmacology.
   b. pharmacodynamics.
   c. pharmacokinetics.
   d. pharmacotherapeutics.
2. **The investigation of the metabolic distribution and absorption of a given drug is known as**
   a. pharmacology.
   b. pharmacodynamics.
   c. pharmacokinetics.
   d. pharmacotherapeutics.
3. **Which of the following pathogens usually do not require the use of antibiotics?**
   a. viruses
   b. bacteria
   c. parasites
   d. fungi
4. **Which of the following drugs is not a bronchodilator?**
   a. epinephrine
   b. acetaminophen
   c. ephedrine
   d. albuterol
5. **Which of the following is used to discourage blood clotting?**
   a. atropine
   b. pseudoephedrine
   c. nitroglycerin
   d. heparin
6. **Common medications used to treat inflammation include all of the following except**
   a. ibuprofen.
   b. acetaminophen.
   c. naproxen.
   d. piroxicam.

7. **Which of the following is not a true statement concerning positive contrast agents?**
   a. A positive contrast agent can be injected into the arterial system.
   b. A positive contrast agent is visualized radiographically as a dark area on a radiograph.
   c. A positive contrast agent usually has a high atomic number.
   d. A positive contrast agent is considered a drug.

8. **Which of the following is not a type of negative contrast?**
   a. oxygen
   b. carbon monoxide
   c. carbon dioxide
   d. nitrous oxide

9. **When choosing the type of water-based contrast to administer, considerations may include which of the following?**
   a. level of osmolarity
   b. type of examination
   c. allergy history of the patient
   d. a and c only
   e. a, b, and c

10. **Within what time period do most contrast reactions occur?**
    a. 30 seconds after injection
    b. 2 minutes after injection
    c. 5 minutes after injection
    d. after a delay

11. **Why should oil-based contrast agents never be injected into the bloodstream?**
    a. They can cause embolism and death.
    b. They are difficult for the liver to metabolize.
    c. They may not be easily excreted by the kidneys.
    d. They usually cause nausea and vomiting.

12. **Which of the following can help to reduce a severe contrast reaction?**
    a. Patients receiving contrast should be well hydrated before contrast is injected.
    b. Proper medical history should be obtained from the patient.
    c. Patients should be aware of possible reactions so that they can notify medical personnel if symptoms occur.
    d. b and c only
    e. a, b, and c

13. **The most common type of contrast used for studies involving the GI system is**
    a. nonionic contrast.
    b. ionic contrast.
    c. barium sulfate.
    d. oil-based contrast.

14. **In which of the following positions should the patient be placed when an enema tip is being inserted?**
    a. lithotomy
    b. Sims'
    c. Trendelenburg
    d. Fowler's

15. **The most common examination that allows visualization of the stomach utilizing contrast is the**
    a. upper GI.
    b. lower GI.
    c. barium enema.
    d. intravenous pyelogram.

16. **Why is it important that a patient not smoke or chew gum prior to a barium enema study?**
    a. It may make the patient nauseous.
    b. It may cause an allergic reaction to the barium.
    c. It causes abdominal cramping.
    d. It may stimulate gastrointestinal secretions.

17. **Which of the following usually requires only a 12-hour patient preparation?**
    a. intravenous pyelogram (IVP)
    b. barium enema (BE)
    c. upper GI (UGI)
    d. a and c only
    e. a and b only
    f. a, b, and c

18. **If BE, IVP, and UGI examinations are to be completed on the same day on the same patient, in what order should they be scheduled?**
    a. IVP, UGI, BE
    b. BE, UGI, IVP
    c. UGI, BE, IVP
    d. IVP, BE, UGI

Appendices

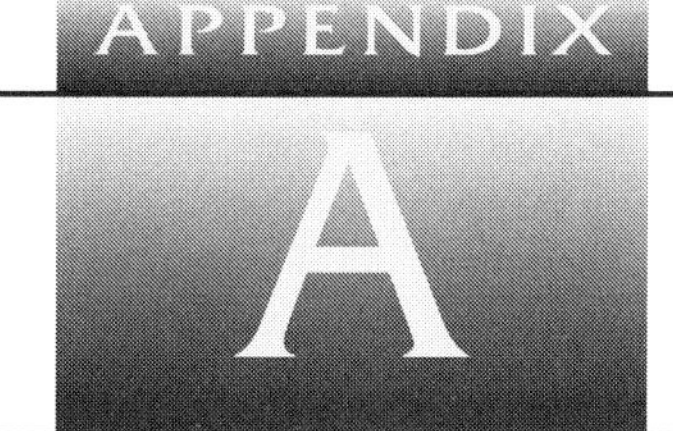

Glossary

Ambulatory Able to move with little assistance.

Anaphylaxis An allergic reaction to an antigen.

Anomaly An abnormality.

Antibody A complex protein produced in response to an antigen.

Antigen A specific protein marker on a cell that identifies the type of cell and may activate the production of antibodies.

Antiseptic Anything that aids in the destruction or repression of microorganisms.

Arrhythmia Irregularity in or absence of rhythm.

Aseptic Free of germs.

Aspiration The entry of gastric contents or fluids into the bronchus and lungs.

Assault An intended threat or harm with or without physical contact.

Bacteria One-celled microorganisms containing both DNA and RNA.

Battery Physical contact without permission.

Body mechanics A system that employs balance, posture, and proper body movement to prevent injury when moving an object or person.

Bradycardia A sluggish pulse rate.

Bradypnea An abnormally slow rate of respiration.

Cardiac arrest A sudden loss of heart function and circulation.

Cardiopulmonary arrest A sudden loss of ventilation and circulation.

Catheter Any tube passing into the body for the purpose of removing or depositing fluid.

Code of ethics A set of principles for a specific practice or profession.

Concussion A shock to the soft tissue of the brain without bruising or laceration.

Contaminate To make unclean, soiled, or unfit for use.

Contraindication Improper or imprudent use or treatment.

Contusion A shock to the brain and soft tissue with bruising.

Cyanosis A condition due to loss of capillary circulation which is characterized by a bluish or grayish skin tone.

Diabetes mellitus A general disorder caused by improper metabolism and inadequate insulin production.

Diastolic Pertaining to diastole; denotes the lowest pressure of the ventricles between heartbeats.

Disinfection The removal of microorganisms by mechanical or chemical means.

Disorientation The inability to identify oneself in relation to time or place.

Distend To stretch or expand.

Dormancy A condition in which the metabolic rate is greatly decreased in order to enable reactivation and continuation.

Dyspnea Difficulty breathing.

Dysrhythmia A condition in which the heart rhythm is abnormal.

Embolus A solid, gas, or liquid mass that obstructs a vessel.

Endoscope A tubelike optical system that allows the observation of organs through a surgical incision or a natural opening.

External respiration A process by which oxygen is delivered to the lungs.

Fomite A substance that clings to and transfers infectious material.

Fowler's A position in which the head of the bed is elevated.

Glasgow Coma Scale A set of standards that can be used to predict a patient's ability and level of recovery from brain injury.

Glucagon A hormone that is naturally secreted by the pancreas; it can be administered by parenteral injection to aid in relaxation of the smooth muscles of the gastrointestinal system.

Heimlich maneuver A technique used to remove an obstructive object from the trachea or pharynx.

Host An organism from which a parasite acquires sustenance.

Hydrate To add or combine with water.

Hyperglycemia A condition caused by a low level of glucose in the blood.

Hypertension Elevated blood pressure.

Hyperventilation An increased rate of respiration and a decreased level of carbon dioxide in the blood.

Hypoglycemia A condition caused by a surplus of glucose in the blood.

Hypotension Decreased blood pressure.

Hypoventilation A decreased rate of respiration and an increased level of carbon dioxide in the blood.

Hypovolemia A sudden decrease in blood volume.

Hypoxia Decreased oxygen in the blood.

Iatrogenic Induced as a result of the effects of medical treatment.

Idiosyncratic A peculiar or unusual individual response.

Immobile Unable to move or to assist in a transfer procedures.

Immune Protected from disease as a result of the production of antibodies or cell-mediated insusceptibility.

Incision A surgical cut or opening.

Incontinence Lack of the ability to maintain bladder or rectal sphincter control.

Incubation The period between exposure and appearance of symptoms.

Infection Invasion and growth of microorganisms which may cause harm to cells and tissues.

Informed consent A procedure that allows patients to make decisions regarding their care based on information provided to them by a health care professional.

Insulin-dependent diabetes A condition resulting from a lack of insulin production.

Internal respiration A process by which oxygen is delivered an carbon dioxide is exchanged in the cells.

Intubate To insert a tube in order to establish or maintain and airway.

Ischemia Death to cells due to lack of circulation.

Isolation A separation for the period of contagiousness.

Lateral Pertaining to either the right or the left side.

Lithotomy position A position in which the patient is lying on her back with her knees bent and legs spread apart.

Lumen The space within a tube or any tubelike structure.

Malpractice Professional misconduct, incompetence, or lack of skill.

MAST pants Medical/military antishock trousers; a garment that restricts the flow of blood to the extremities.

Meatus An opening

Microorganism A microscopic living organism.

Myocardial infarct Blockage of one or more of the pulmonary arteries.

Nasoenteric (NE) tube A tube that is inserted into the nose through the esophagus and into the small bowel.

Nasogastric (NG) tube A tube that is inserted into the nose through the esophagus and into the stomach.

Nebulize To produce a fine mist or spray in which the particles are very small.

Negative contrast Radiographic contrast that appears radiolucent.

Nosocomial Anything that occurs within the health care environment.

Oxyhemoglobin A combined form of hemoglobin and oxygen encountered in arterial blood.

Paralysis A temporary or permanent loss of movement or function.

Paraplegia Paralysis from the waist down.

Parenteral Any route of drug administration other than via the gastrointestinal system.

Pathogen A disease-causing microorganism.

Percutaneous Accomplished by going through the skin

Permeable Allows the passage of fluid.

Phagocyte Any cell having the ability to destroy or consume another cell.

Pharmacodynamics A branch of science that studies the specific effects of a drug.

Pharmacokinetics A branch of science that investigates the metabolic and absorption processes of specific drugs within the body.

Pharmacology A branch of science that studies drugs and their uses, composition, and interaction.

Pleura A lining that surrounds the lung.

Pneumothorax A collection of air outside the lung, usually within the pleural space.

Positive contrast Radiographic contrast that appears radioopaque.

Prone Lying flat on the abdomen.

Pulmonary embolism Blockage of the pulmonary artery as the result of a thrombus.

Pulse The rate at which the walls of the heart contract to push blood through the arteries.

Pulse oximeter A device used to measure oxygen saturation in the blood.

Quadriplegia Paralysis from the neck down.

Radiolucent An area that is easily penetrated by x rays and appears dark on a radiograph.

Radioopaque Describes an area that is impenetrable to x rays and appears light on a radiograph.

Reflux Backward flow.

Respiration A process in which the body exchanges oxygen and carbon dioxide.

Respiratory distress A condition in which there is severe inadequacy of the lungs in oxygenating the blood.

Respiratory failure A condition, either acute or chronic, in which the lungs fail to oxygenate the blood.

Resuscitate To revive after evident death.

Scope of practice Defines specific responsibilities within a health care profession.

Secretion A substance composed of certain types of body fluids.

Seizure Sudden convulsion, loss of consciousness, motor, or sensory function due to brain dysfunction.

Sims' A position in which a patient is placed in the left lateral position with the right knee bent and drawn toward the abdomen.

Slide board A long board, usually made of hard plastic, that is used to aid in patient movement.

Sphygmomanometer A device used to indirectly measure arterial blood pressure.

Spore A specific cell that enables pathogens to resist harsh environmental influences.

Sterilize A procedure that renders something free of living organisms.

Stethoscope An instrument that conveys sounds produced in the body.

Stroke A sudden loss of cognizance as the result of a brain hemorrhage, thrombus, or embolus.

Subarachnoid Below the arachnoid membrane which covers the brain.

Suction To reduce air pressure, or the action of suck-up.

Supine Lying flat on one's back.

Suture Surgical stitching material, or the process of joining with surgical stitching.

Syncope A brief loss of consciousness due to a lack of blood flow to the brain.

Systolic Pertaining to systole; denotes the force with which the heart contracts.

Tachycardia A rapid pulse rate.

Tachypnea Rapid respiration.

Thermometer A device used to measure the degree of heat or cold.

Thrombus A blood clot.

Tort A civil wrong involving an individual or private property; may be an intentional or an unintentional act.

Toxicity Measurement or amount of poison.

Trauma A physical or emotional injury caused by oneself or by an outside source.

Trauma team A group of professionals trained to handle specific acute care situations usually related to physical trauma.

Trendelenburg A variation of the supine position in which the patient's feet are elevated and the head is lowered.

Unconscious Without awareness of one's surroundings or environment.

Vasodilation Dilation of the vessels.

Venipuncture Puncture of a vein.

Ventricular fibrillation A condition due to the absence of systematic pumping of blood in the ventricles which may lead to lack of proper blood flow to the brain and death.

Appropriate Textbooks

deWitt S. Rambo's Nursing Skills for Clinical Practice, 4th ed. WB Saunders, Philadelphia, 1994.

Gould B. Pathophysiology for the Health-Related Professions. WB Saunders, Philadelphia, 1997.

Kowalczyk N, Donnett K. Integrated Patient Care for the Imaging Professional. Mosby–Year Book, St. Louis, 1996.

Meeker MR, Rothrock JC. Alexander's Care of the Patient in Surgery, 10th ed. Mosby–Year Book, St. Louis, 1995.

Taber CW. Taber's Cyclopedic Medical Dictionary. FA Davis, Philadelphia, 1997.

Torres LS. Basic Medical Techniques and Patient Care in Imaging Technology, 5th ed. Lippincott–Raven, Philadelphia, 1997.

Tortorici M. Administration of Imaging Pharmaceuticals. WB Saunders, Philadelphia, 1996.

Tucker SM, Canobbie MM, Paquette EV, Wells MF. Patient Care Standards, 6th ed. Mosby–Year Book, St. Louis, 1996.

Wilson BJ. Ethics and Basic Law for Medical Imaging Professionals. F.A. Davis, Philadelphia, 1997.

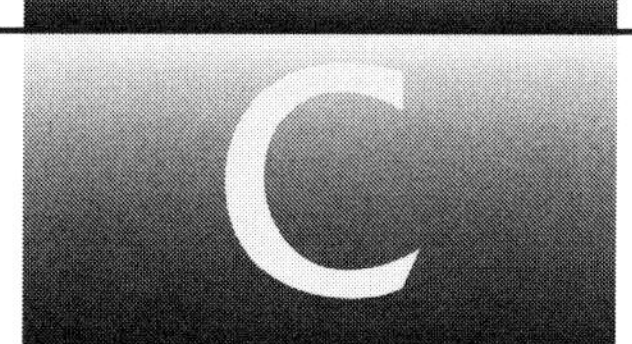

Answers

Chapter 1
1. d
2. c
3. a
4. d
5. a
6. b
7. c
8. a
9. c
10. b
11. a
12. d
13. a
14. c
15. d

Chapter 2
1. a
2. c
3. b
4. b
5. c
6. c
7. d
8. b
9. b
10. a
11. c
12. b

Chapter 3
1. c
2. d
3. b
4. c
5. d
6. d
7. b
8. c
9. d
10. b
11. c
12. a
13. d
14. d
15. b
16. b
17. a
18. a

Chapter 4
1. a
2. d
3. c
4. b
5. b
6. c
7. d
8. d
9. b
10. a
11. d
12. b
13. b
14. c
15. c
16. a
17. a
18. b
19. c
20. a

Chapter 5
1. b
2. c
3. b
4. d
5. d
6. b
7. c
8. d
9. d
10. b
11. b
12. d
13. a
14. c
15. d
16. a
17. c
18. c
19. a
20. b

Chapter 6
1. c
2. b
3. a
4. b
5. b
6. c
7. d
8. b
9. a
10. a
11. a
12. e
13. c
14. b
15. b
16. c
17. d
18. d
19. b
20. d

Chapter 7
1. b
2. c
3. a
4. c
5. d
6. c
7. a
8. d
9. c
10. d
11. c
12. a
13. c
14. b
15. b
16. d
17. d
18. d

Chapter 8
1. a
2. b
3. c
4. d
5. a
6. b
7. b
8. d
9. e
10. b
11. b
12. c

Chapter 9
1. a
2. c
3. d
4. d
5. a
6. b
7. e
8. a
9. c
10. b
11. c
12. c
13. d
14. c
15. b
16. a

Chapter 10
1. a
2. b

3. c
4. d
5. b
6. a
7. c
8. b
9. b
10. d
11. d
12. a

Chapter 11

1. b
2. c
3. a
4. b
5. a
6. b
7. b
8. b
9. e
10. c
11. a
12. e
13. c
14. b
15. a
16. d
17. d
18. d

Notes

ISBN 0-07-070632-8
90000
9 780070 706323

WILLIAMS: PATIENT CARE